diet
starts
m✕nday

WELBECK
BALANCE

diet starts mxnday

DITCH the scales, RECLAIM your body & LIVE LIFE to the full

LAURA ADLINGTON

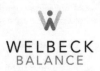

WELBECK
BALANCE

Published in 2024 by Welbeck Balance
An imprint of Welbeck Non-Fiction Limited
Part of Welbeck Publishing Group
Offices in: London – 20 Mortimer Street, London W1T 3JW &
Sydney – Level 17, 207 Kent St, Sydney NSW 2000 Australia
www.welbeckpublishing.com

A CIP catalogue record for this book is available from the British Library.

ISBN
Hardback – 978-1-80129-297-9

Typeset by Lapiz Digital Services
Printed and bound in Great Britain by Clays Ltd Elcograf S.p.A.

10 9 8 7 6 5 4 3 2 1

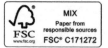

Note/Disclaimer
Welbeck encourages and welcomes diversity and different viewpoints. However, all
views, thoughts, and opinions expressed in this book are the author's own and are not
necessarily representative of Welbeck Publishing Group as an organization. Welbeck
Publishing Group makes no representations or warranties of any kind, express or implied,
with respect to the accuracy, completeness, suitability or currency of the contents of this
book, and specifically disclaims, to the extent permitted by law, any implied warranties
of merchantability or fitness for a particular purpose and any injury, illness, damage,
death, liability or loss incurred, directly or indirectly from the use or application of any
of the information contained in this book. This book is solely intended for informational
purposes and guidance only and is not intended to replace, diagnose, treat or act as a
substitute for professional and expert medical and/or psychiatric advice. The author and
the publisher are not medical practitioners nor counsellors and professional advice should
be sought before embarking on any health-related programme.

Any names, characters, trademarks, service marks and trade names detailed in
this book are the property of their respective owners and are used solely for
identification and reference purposes. This book is a publication of Welbeck
Non-Fiction Ltd, part of Welbeck Publishing Group and has not been licensed,
approved, sponsored or endorsed by any person or entity.

Every reasonable effort has been made to trace copyright holders of material
produced in this book, but if any have been inadvertently overlooked
the publishers would be glad to hear from them.

Contents

Introduction

Hello! I'm so pleased you've picked up this book.

Welcome to *Diet Starts Monday*. In case you were in any doubt, the title is obviously completely ironic.

I spent years hearing phrases like this and listening to the women around me – funny, kind, intelligent women – talk about how much they needed to lose weight and what new diet they were on (maybe you did too). And do you know what? I found it so fucking boring. We are SO much more than what we look like and the size of our jeans.

So this is NOT a book about how to stick to a diet, or about putting off your diet until next week.

This is a book that wants you to bin diet culture for good. To never say "Diet starts Monday" EVER again.

To stop finding your worth as a person in a number on a set of scales or the label in a dress.

To reclaim your body, in all its jiggly glory, from the clutches of the diet and fitness industries.

And to live a life that makes you happy.

ABOUT THIS BOOK

Diet Starts Monday is the book I wish I had growing up.

Full of personal stories, my hope is that it will not only empower you but also help you make peace with what you see in the mirror.

For too long we, as women, have been made to feel as if we have no choice but to remain trapped in the hamster wheel of body hate and dieting. And I'm here to tell you, quite simply, that you *don't*.

Throughout these pages, I will share the realities of what it's like being in a bigger body, why we've been conditioned to fear the word "fat" and how hard it is to take up space in a world that wants to shrink you. I'll also be calling out the societal pressures to be something we're not and discussing the many pitfalls of diet culture.

While I talk a lot about my own experiences as a plus-size woman, my aim is to help you find self-acceptance (and maybe even self-love) whether you're a size 6 or 36, able-bodied or disabled, young or old. *Diet Starts Monday* is for everyone.

HOW TO GET THE MOST OUT OF
DIET STARTS MONDAY

Diet Starts Monday is divided into two parts, and I recommend you read each part through in order.

In Part One, we'll be "Unpacking the Problem" – looking to understand WHY we, as women, have been made to feel like we're never good enough (thank you, diet culture, the media and toxic beauty standards!).

This will include exploring ever-changing beauty standards through the years, and the huge impact of weight stigma and diet culture.

Then, in Part Two, we'll be "Taking Back the Power" by looking at HOW you can start living a full, fulfilling and happy life in the body you are in RIGHT NOW.

And I'll be honest here: it *does* take some work. We'll explore topics such as body neutrality, finding joy in movement and intuitive eating. I'm really excited to share with you what I've learnt (and am still learning) on the road to self-acceptance.

Peppered throughout the book are lots of research stats from a range of informed sources, and words of wisdom from leaders in relevant fields – from medicine and psychotherapy to nutrition and fitness. I also had the pleasure of chatting with some of my favourite experts, and am so grateful I've been able to include their invaluable knowledge in this book.

I spoke with NHS doctor and nutritionist Dr Joshua Wolrich on the relationship between weight and health, inclusive personal trainer Tally Rye on exercise and movement, body positivity campaigner Molly Forbes on breaking the intergenerational cycle of diet culture, relationship expert Michelle Elman on dating in a plus-size body and knowing your worth, body-image advocate Stephanie Yeboah on the nuances of body positivity and the Fat Acceptance Movement and clinical psychologist Dr Emma Cotterill on the effects our body image can have on our mental health and wellbeing.

You'll also find practical "Self-Empowerment Tasks" in each chapter – designed to help you reflect on and overcome your own body image struggles. There's a big difference between understanding something on a *conscious* level and internalising it so that you actually *feel* differently about yourself, so it's important that you do the tasks as well as read the book.

My hope is that the combination of all of this will help to provide you with a grounded but inspiring framework for changing the way you view yourself and ending the yo-yo diet cycle once and for all.

Is *Diet Starts Monday* a magical cure-all? Absolutely not. But I hope you learn from it and maybe even pick it up again any time you need reminding that the way you look is the least interesting thing about you.

PART 1

UNPACKING THE PROBLEM

The messages telling us that our bodies are the problem are everywhere: on TV, on social media and in magazines. They're also in our homes, in the workplace and in the playground.

But the good news is that, once you know what the problem is, it's a lot easier to find the solution.

In this first part of the book, I'm going to help you with this by shining a light on all the ways you've been made to feel bad about yourself and the way you look.

1

"Such a pretty face"
My big fat life so far

I was eight years old when I was put on my first diet.

It all started after a visit to my nan's house, during which she told me I shouldn't be wearing the dress I had on because I was "getting chubby". After that, talk of eating less and moving more floated around our house a lot, but nothing seemed to curb my appetite and, at 11 years old, I was much bigger than all the kids in my school and being badly bullied for it.

On the last day of primary school, all of my classmates were signing each other's T-shirts and I remember one kid, Sean, writing the word "FAT" in great big capital letters across my entire back in permanent marker. I know, what a prick.

Even at that young age, I remember being very aware of my body, its bigness, and the problem that people around me often seemed to have with that. I realised that my body wasn't considered normal, and that, in one way or another, I was being judged. I didn't just have a body; I *was* my body.

One summer, my dad decided it would be a good idea for us all to get on the scales, so we could lose weight together, "as a family". He was more than a little surprised by the weight he saw when I stepped on, and let out a jarring and audible gasp of astonishment that made my stomach do a little flip-flop. Shame ate away at me, and my cheeks turned pink at the sense of disapproval and embarrassment that I felt. It was as if I'd failed a test I didn't even know I'd taken.

I burst into tears, ran out of the house and made a beeline for the tent my brother and I had set up in the garden – partly because I wanted to get as far away from my dad, and the rest of the family, as physically possible, but *mainly* because I knew we had a stash of Wagon Wheels hidden under the mountain of sleeping bags and blankets.

I can laugh about it now, but I remember crying my little heart out as I stuffed them all into my mouth at speed; a mixture of chocolate, snot and tears stained my face like a modern-day Bruce Bogtrotter. Little did I know that would be the start of a lifelong battle with binge-eating and secret eating.

Over the years I regularly squirrelled away chocolate and other sweet treats in my bedroom so that I could eat them in private whenever I got the urge. There was something about the deceit, the sugar and the solitude that made it all the more appealing.

The more a certain food was off limits, the more I wanted it. But of course, after each binge would come the familiar feelings of guilt and shame, followed by the voice in my head saying, "Ugh, I hate myself. *Why* did I do that?"

MY FIRST FORAY INTO THE WORLD OF DIETING

When I was 13, I weighed around 14 stone (196 lb/89 kg) and wore a UK size 16 (US 20). My parents were so concerned that they decided it was time for an intervention, and that's when my mum took me to my first Slimming World group.

It's funny how insignificant things stick in your head, isn't it? I can still picture the room the meeting was held in, every Wednesday night – in the upstairs function room of our local pub. It was huge and had an ugly, floral, red carpet that stank of stale booze and cigarettes, which they'd tried (unsuccessfully) to mask with cheap air freshener.

At the far end of the room, in front of the tall bay windows, was a row of helpers all lined up to weigh us or sell us something. It started with the scales – or the "sad step", as I now like to call it – and was followed by the magazines, "healthy" snack bars and raffle tickets you felt obliged to buy.

I remember shame creeping in as I stood on the scales for the first time and the lady wrote down my weight in my starter pack. She commented to my mum that I had "such a pretty face", which was, of course, code for "She'd be so much prettier if she wasn't such a fat bastard".

Once everyone had weighed in, we sat in a semi-circle like the kind you see in group therapy scenes on TV shows. Our group leader, Beryl, would go around the room each week, noting everyone's achievements (or lack there of). "You've put on a pound this week, Sheila. What happened? You were so *good* last week!?"

I'll never forget the woman who was congratulated for losing 6 pounds (2.7 kg) in a week, even though it was because she had diarrhoea. "Every cloud!" quipped Beryl.

One person was at their "target weight" and a few women were losing weight, but the vast majority were really struggling to shift more than a pound, if that, each week. They often spoke about their lack of willpower, which, when I think about it now, makes me really sad. But what struck me the most was the quest by all of them to be thin. Not healthy, but thin.

Many of the women spoke about how they hated their bodies, and I remember one lady (who was half the size I was and double my age), telling us all how she resembled a fat whale. "I just feel like a failure," she said. "Like I've let myself go."

This was a real coming-of-age moment for me. It taught me that my body was something to be judged and feared, that I was somehow a failure as a person in my current "fat" form, and that a life in a body like mine was no life at all.

Another thing these weekly weigh-ins "taught" me was that certain foods were "sinful" or "bad". Food wasn't there to fuel us or, god forbid, enjoy. Food, according to Slimming World and every other diet club I've since encountered, was laden with a lot of moral connotations: it was either "good" or "bad", and I was therefore either "good" or "bad" for eating it.

Not knowing any different, and with everyone around me saying the same kind of things, I just presumed this was how things had to be. So, eager to please, I did what I was told. I was willing to do anything to be "fixed", i.e. to be skinny.

I was elated when I lost 8 pounds (3.6 kg) in my first week. I lost a fair amount in subsequent weeks too – enough for the people around me to notice and congratulate me. I even remember being cat-called in the street, which, looking back, was disgusting because I was still in my school uniform. But I can't lie, it made me feel attractive for the first time in my life, and it was nice.

People were definitely kinder to me when I was smaller. The world felt like a safer place. "Wow, is this what life is like for 'normal' people?" I would think to myself. "Is this what freedom feels like?"

At the start of the diet and for a couple of months after, I fixated on what life would be like when I eventually got down to my target weight. I would think of all the friends I'd have, all the parties I'd get invited to, all the boys I'd kiss, and all the lovely clothes from Tammy Girl or Topshop I would finally be able to fit into. "This is it!" I'd say to myself. "Laura version 2.0 will be happier, prettier, more successful, more loveable, more fashionable. Slimmer. Better. THIS IS IT!" I was a walking "before" photo.

But 14-year-old Laura very quickly got bored of meat-free and carb-free days, and not eating much on weigh-in days and the days leading up to them.

I got bored of not eating McDonald's on a Saturday, like everyone else was. I got tired of having salad for my lunch instead of sandwiches. I got frustrated with being punished for wanting to just enjoy food – something that felt so natural to me.

And, as a result, any opportunity to eat the foods I loved became an opportunity to overindulge, often to the point of feeling unwell. Chips, chocolate, cake and crisps brought me unparalleled joy. They were unrivalled in their ability to make me euphorically happy, even if fleetingly.

To me, food was like a drug. I would think about it constantly and wonder when, and what, I'd eat next. And just like a drug addict, I didn't want to give it up.

After a while, I followed the Slimming World plan less and less, and the weight losses stalled. I felt frustrated and ashamed. "Why can't I just eat what I want and be skinny like my brother? Like all the girls in my class? What is *wrong* with me?"

I came up with excuse after excuse to stop going to the Slimming World meetings, until my parents eventually caved in and let me give it up altogether.

But, while I knew I couldn't continue with the diet, I also knew there was no way I was going to be "allowed" to be in a body that wasn't the "right" size, as it had been made clear to me from such a young age that being fat was "bad" …

BODY-CONSCIOUS FROM A YOUNG AGE

Like a lot of people, I grew up in a household obsessed with appearances and totally consumed by the belief that weight was equal to worth. My mum was constantly on a diet, and my dad was always on at me to go on one (while at the same time always telling me I had to clear my plate).

We would also get rewarded for good behaviour with "nice" food and punished by a lack of it. If we'd been good, we'd go out for a meal or get a takeaway, and if we'd been bad, we weren't allowed dessert or treats. I know this isn't unique, but I think in our house, it was just a bit more extreme. Food was used as a way to show love and affection, and, because my mum grew up with a lack of both, she wanted to give it to my brother and me in spades. "What's that darling, you want a packet of Skittles for breakfast? Sure, go ahead!"

When I packed in Slimming World and put on all the weight I'd lost, my dad sat me down one day and told me no one will ever love me "looking like that". "Men will sleep with you," he said. "But they won't stick around." I was 15.

My dad and I are best friends now, but it still stings when I think about it. And I'd be lying if I said it didn't have a big effect on my relationship with food (and my relationships in general) for years after.

A huge chunk of my life, from the age of about eight to well into my late 20s, involved weathering the storm of conversations about my body. I lived in almost constant fear of family members passing comment on what I was eating, which meant that it was really only on special occasions like birthdays and Christmases where I felt free to eat what I wanted and not be called out for it.

In every other respect, I had a wonderful childhood. I felt loved, protected, safe and happy. But I also felt defined – and trapped – by my weight. It was a vicious circle: the more weight I gained, the more I would seek comfort in food, and the more I sought comfort in food, the more weight I would gain.

I think I also grew up a lot quicker than most people because when you're bigger, you often look older, and, as such, you get treated that way. You also learn to grow a thick skin and think of other ways to be seen as a worthy human.

For me, this meant things like being the "funny one", the "caring one", the one with the nicest handbag, the hyper feminine one in the pretty dress – a practice known in the fat-liberation movement as being the "good fatty", which you'll read more about in Chapter 8.

I often wonder what my life would have been like if my size hadn't been put under the spotlight so much and if I hadn't always been made to feel like the black sheep. Would I still be fat? Would I be less fat? Would I feel more "successful", more likeable, more loveable?

I also can't help but wonder how different my life might have been if someone, anyone, would have just said to me, "Hey, it's OK to be bigger than your friends. Some people are just built differently."

I honestly don't blame my mum and dad. I know in my heart that they did the best they could and, like most parents, they had my best interests at heart. I also have to acknowledge the fact there wasn't really any advice back then on how to raise a fat kid.

These days, we all have a mutual respect and understanding that we don't talk about my weight. But it took a long time (and a long list of unsuccessful diets) to get to this point.

COULD SURGERY BE THE "MAGIC CURE"?

Throughout my late teens and 20s, I started on countless attempts to lose weight. I tried everything from the Dukan diet and the detox diet to keto and Cambridge. I would start every one with the eagerness of a new puppy ready to be let off its leash for the first time. But the end result was always the same: I simply couldn't sustain the intense restriction and I'd always put the weight back on.

I would ditch the diet, binge-eat and gain even more weight until the feelings of "I hate myself. I'm a monster. I have to do something about this" settled in hard enough for me to embark on the next one.

I look back now at the time (and money) I spent on these fad diets and feel incredibly sad. I knew I needed help to overcome what felt like an addiction to food, but, no matter where I looked, I just couldn't find it.

I felt angry at the lack of support. Not just for me, but for other people like me, too. It bothered me that people with recognised eating disorders, such as anorexia and bulimia, were met with what felt like endless amounts of sympathy, as well as specialist doctors and clinics, whereas it was years before binge-eating disorder was categorised by medical professionals. And even then, all it felt like we got was a telling off and a marching to the nearest Weight Watchers group.

As a result, at the time, it seemed to me that my only option to rid myself of this extra weight once and for all was to have weight-loss (bariatric) surgery. I'd toyed with the idea of having a gastric band (a form of bariatric surgery) for years – thinking it would, at last, be the magic cure that solved all my problems. But it wasn't until I hit 30 that I went to my GP to discuss having one.

My (now) husband and I had been trying for a baby for several years with no luck, and the pain of infertility was excruciating. We'd had to fight for over a year just to have the most basic fertility tests; they wouldn't initially give us tests, as they said that even if they came back showing something was wrong, they wouldn't be able to offer us fertility treatment due to our BMIs (body mass index) not being below 30. I'll never forget the specialist telling me I had to lose 14 stone (196 lb/89 kg) in order to even be considered a candidate for IVF. My world fell apart in that moment, and all my hopes of holding a baby – my baby – in my arms, felt futile. "This is it!" I told myself. "I'm going to have bariatric surgery, lose the weight and have a baby. This is what I have to do."

I was on the waiting list for about a year. There were several hoops I had to jump through to prove my eligibility – mainly pointless meetings with people who had no idea of the struggles I was facing, or what life was like being in a body like mine. In the year leading up to the surgery, I didn't buy any new clothes – not even a new pair of knickers, because I had such high hopes of soon filling my wardrobe with smaller ones.

In my final assessment, my doctor laid out all the things I was in store for:

1. Only being able to eat meals the size of an egg for the rest of my life
2. Being at risk of severe complications, including death
3. A high chance of depression (as experienced by a lot of patients who no longer have food as a source of joy and comfort)
4. Addiction replacement (a lot of patients have been found to swap their addiction with alcohol, drugs and/or gambling)
5. Having to take a plethora of different vitamins for the rest of my life

It makes me laugh when people say bariatric surgery is the easy option. I don't think anyone could honestly read the above and say that. But, despite all the risks, I decided I wanted to go ahead with it anyway.

Because of my high BMI, I was told that a gastric bypass was the only option for me. Gastric bands were apparently "not in vogue" because you could "cheat" them with high-calorie, liquified foods like ice cream, and lots of patients regained the weight they lost. With the bypass, my stomach would be cut to a third of its size, and then rerouted to my large intestine. This was so that a) I wouldn't be able to eat as much, and b) I wouldn't absorb the calories from the food I did eat.

I was dead set on going ahead with it all, right up until two weeks before the operation, when I had to go on something called a Liver Reduction

Diet, or LRD for short. This meant eating around 300 to 500 calories a day for my liver to shrink enough for the surgeon to access my stomach.

The first week was intense and I was, of course, very hungry and very grumpy. I'm not really sure what changed after week one; it wasn't one particular lightbulb moment that made me think "I can't do this", but doubt definitely started to creep in by the time I got to week two. I began to fear the operating table, the inevitable (and other potential) side effects, as well as not being able to enjoy a proper meal with my family or friends ever again.

The hunger and fear got too much and, three days before the surgery, I went to my local petrol station and bought a mountain of "bad" food and stuffed it down my face. I'm not proud of this. In fact, to this day, I'm quite embarrassed about it. But, in that moment, I was able to admit to myself what I think I knew deep down already: that the surgery wasn't right for me, because stapling my stomach wasn't going to heal my relationship with food. Years of disordered eating weren't suddenly going to be resolved overnight by a knife and some staples.

My decision not to have the surgery was met with mixed emotions from my loved ones. Some were relieved, others were disappointed. Feelings of guilt and shame consumed my brain for a long time after, but I told myself (and everyone else) that I would still "lose the weight", just in a healthier, more sensible way. But, surprise, surprise, I didn't ...

A SHIFT IN MINDSET

For as long as I could remember, I had always thought (or been led to believe) that I had to be on a diet (or at least *talking* about going on one) – like a "good fatty". But, a while after making the decision to reject the surgery, I began to wonder what my life would be like if I no longer obsessed about "getting skinny". "Would it really be such a bad thing to stay at the size I was?" I started to ask myself.

Then, that very same year – in 2020, when I was 30 – my life completely changed, and not just because of Covid.

My passion for baking had won me a spot as a baker on a TV show called *The Great British Bake Off*. It felt amazing to be part of a show I'd loved for so many years. (I remember racing home from work on a Tuesday night via the shops to pick up supplies so I could bake along with whatever the theme of the week was.)

In truth, I never thought I stood a chance of getting on the show, but, to my surprise, I kept getting through the various audition stages. When they called me and told me I was going to be one of the 12 bakers, I couldn't believe it. But it wasn't long before my excitement turned to concern. What will people say about a fat bird baking on telly? Am I cut out to handle it?

When the filming had wrapped, there was a short wait until the show was live, and, on the day the bakers of 2020 were publicly announced, a lot of the tabloids ran stories on us. I remember someone sending me a link to an article run by my local newspaper. The theme of the article was your standard "Local girl does good", so, full of optimism, I decided to look at the comments. The first one read: "Looks like someone's been eating all the practice bakes …" And the second one read: "And everyone else's". Oof! That hit me hard. This was just the announcement, and I was already getting abuse. I wish I could say they were the only nasty comments I received, but sadly it was the start of many.

Because I'd learnt how to develop a thick skin from a young age (as I mentioned earlier – you have to when you grow up different), most of the vitriol I got was water off a duck's back – partly because I was used to receiving abuse, and partly because of the hundreds, eventually thousands, of messages of support from other women who finally saw themselves represented on TV and felt a connection to me and my story.

In the years leading to that point, I had felt completely alone with my body-image struggles – a "fat freak" who had no self-discipline and would never be able to make peace with her body. But how wrong I had been all that time about being *alone* in the way I was feeling.

From the very first episode, I started to hear from women all over the world who had struggled, or were still struggling, with their weight and self-worth. And it made me realise that we all have body issues and hang-ups, no matter our size. You can be a size 6 or 36 and still grapple with thoughts of not liking your stomach, your legs, your cellulite, your scar, your big nose or your acne-prone skin.

This realisation led me down a rabbit hole of research into diet culture, beauty standards, the body positivity movement, obesity studies and everything body-image related. In 2022, I started a podcast about body confidence called *Go Love Yourself*, and I started to curate my social media feed more mindfully (see Chapter 8 for more on this). I also started wearing colour instead of black, and saying yes to new experiences instead of always turning them down. And I realised, after years of feeling like a failure, that it wasn't my fault that the diets hadn't worked, and, most importantly, that my weight wasn't equal to my worth.

I finally learned that no matter my size, I was worthy of love and respect, just like everyone else.

While the feeling of wanting Laura version 2.0 still pops up every now and again, I can honestly say that, as I'm writing this, I'm the heaviest I've ever been and I'm also the happiest.

I'd be lying if I said I didn't still want to be smaller at times – because I know my life would be easier if I was – but I've come to accept myself for who I am now, instead of constantly wanting to change. And that's why I think this book is so important.

WHATEVER YOUR STORY, YOU'RE NOT ALONE

I want to show you how wrong it is that we, as women, have been made to feel like we "should" look a certain way and therefore always be on a diet, and prove to you that it *is* possible to have a healthier relationship with food and exercise – as well as a better body image – without dieting.

I want to make you see that your body has never been the problem.

The way I see it, you have two options:

- You can yo-yo diet for the rest of your life, with the potential to be miserable and feel like your body – and life – are temporary.
- *Or* you can accept who you are, make peace with food and live the fullest, happiest life you can – *now*.

And no, that doesn't mean I'm advocating for us all to eat 40 donuts a day and sit on the sofa the whole time. But I *am* advocating for us to shift the focus to health instead of weight, to stop being slaves to diets and to stop worrying about every roll, every stretch mark and every wrinkle.

Your story might be completely different to mine – it may be that you've gained weight in later life, are struggling to come to terms with your body after having a child (or multiple children), or that you have a disability. You might be smaller than me or bigger than me. Whatever your story, my hope is that some of the experience that I've gained over the years, and that I share within this book, will resonate with you and make you feel less alone.

I want you to know that it really is possible to make peace with what you see in the mirror, just as you are. It is *not* your life's purpose to lose weight. And you were *not* put on this Earth to look like a Victoria's Secret model. No one is going to stand up at your funeral and say, "She had a great thigh gap and wore size 8 jeans." It's time to educate ourselves, take back the power, reclaim our bodies and live life to the full.

SELF-EMPOWERMENT TASK

As I mentioned earlier, throughout this book there will be tasks for you to complete in each chapter. So, grab a notebook or a journal, and let's get you going on your journey of making peace with your body – for good.

To start, take a little time out for yourself and write a letter to your body. You might want to apologise to her for all those times you didn't honour her, to thank her for everything she's done for you and to let her know that you're now ready to be kinder to her. Open your heart and write down what you've always thought, but never said.

On the next page is a letter I wrote mine, to give you an example. Writing it was extremely cathartic.

Dear body,

It feels strange writing a letter to you. I've spent so much of my life hating you, judging you, feeling betrayed by you and trying to make you something you were never meant to be.

So, I want to start by saying ... I'm sorry.

I'm sorry for all the times I neglected you, abused you, ignored you. For all the times I've felt ashamed of you, compared you to others and wished you were different. And for all the times I've looked at you with disgust and frustration, measuring your value in only pounds and inches.

I'm sorry for all the names I called you. And for all the prodding and poking and sucking in.

In my attempt to gain control over you, I've subjected you to everything from strict diets and starvation, to punishing workouts and thoughts you'd be better off dead.

For the longest time I resented you. I wanted to take scissors to parts of you and cut them off, because you made me feel like a prisoner in my own skin.

I've resented you for not looking like the people I saw on the magazine covers and, most importantly, for not enabling me to be the one thing I always wanted to be: a mother.

If I'm being honest, I think I will always resent you for that.

But, I also want to acknowledge all that you have done for me and say thank you for carrying me through each day, each challenge and each triumph.

Thank you for protecting me, and for giving me the freedom to move through, and experience, this world.

I'm ready to listen to you now.

Yours,
Laura

2

Fearing the "F" word
The power of three letters

I was at a friend's 30th birthday party recently, chatting to a woman I had just met about her life and her kids, when she asked me what I did for a living. I told her about my work in the body-confidence and plus-size fashion space (the term "plus size" being used to categorise anyone that's bigger than a UK size 18, or US size 14).

I started to share my frustrations with the industry and the lack of fashionable clothes for plus-size women, when she turned to me and said, "Oh, I know exactly how you feel. When I was pregnant and suddenly grew these big boobs, I couldn't find anything to fit my size 8 frame. It was a nightmare."

"Try being fat," I retorted, half joking, half annoyed at her lack of awareness.

"Oh, don't say that," she replied. "You're not fat, you're beautiful."

What I wanted to say was "Bitch, I'm both." But, instead, I thanked her, made my excuses and walked away.

This slightly clumsy interaction didn't offend me at all, but it definitely got me thinking about the word "fat" and how, for such a small word, it holds such immense power.

In this chapter, we're going to look at how and why we've been conditioned to fear the word "fat" and, most importantly, how we can reclaim it, so it no longer hurts us.

FATPHOBIA AND ANTI-FAT BIAS

Sometimes it feels like the worst thing you can be in this world is fat. From a very young age, we're taught that fat is bad and thin is good, and that having a fat body should be avoided at all costs. This lesson gets passed down from generation to generation, and it's been woven so tightly into our subconscious that we often don't even question it.

Remember when we were told Bridget Jones was fat when she weighed only 9 1/2 stone (130 lb/60 kg)? Or when the world collectively fat-shamed Jessica Simpson for gaining weight in her Daisy Duke era, when, in reality, she was probably only a UK size 12 (US size 8)?

From the time I was eight up until about the age of 30, I honestly thought hating my body was just part of being a woman. *"Aren't we always supposed to be on a diet and criticising our bodies?"* Like a lot of women, I always felt like I was on a treadmill, chasing a dangling carrot that was just. out. of. reach. And it was exhausting.

Our culture is, undoubtedly, fixated on "fixing" fatness – and I *really* dislike the narrative that fat people need to be fixed.

As a society, we suffer from a collective, internalised fatphobia that does a lot more harm than good. Fatphobia is defined as the "irrational fear of, aversion to, or discrimination against, obesity, or people with obesity". I think fatphobia exists because – despite a lot of evidence to the contrary – there is still a belief that fatness is an individual failing, and one that can (and must be) controlled.

Sometimes fatphobia is glaringly obvious – such as in the ads for Weight Watchers ("Inside every overweight woman is the woman she knows she can be" – Oprah) and in the magazine articles about how to get a bikini-worthy body. ("Do a detox! Carbs are the enemy!") But more often than not, it's subtle. It's the "I'm just concerned about your health", or the casual, judgemental glance at someone's shopping basket in the confectionery aisle, with the unspoken "Should you be eating that?" written all over their face.

Fat activist and author Aubrey Gordon (also known as Your Fat Friend) likens fatphobia to air pollution. "Some days we see it, other days we don't," she says. "But we still breathe it in." In recent years, however, Gordon has moved away from using the word "fatphobia" and instead prefers the term "anti-fat bias". She says that using the term "phobia" to describe discriminatory attitudes can be both confusing and stigmatising for mental health, as it implies a fear of fatness or fat people, when this is not always the case. Many people who hold "anti-fat" attitudes actively dislike or hate fat people, so she believes describing this as a phobia normalises harmful behaviour towards fat people.

THE LAST ACCEPTABLE FORM OF PREJUDICE

Whether you prefer the term fatphobia or anti-fat bias, one thing I'm sure we can all agree on is that they need to be given the middle finger.

Fat-shaming can sometimes feel like the last acceptable form of prejudice. Any public display of racism, sexism or homophobia are, correctly, met with intense criticism and harsh consequences. Yet derogatory comments or jokes about fat people still seem to be fair game in certain environments.

I think this is because of the archaic view that fatness is a choice – that we are lazy and stupid, and simply need to "eat less, move more". Being fat is also often associated with poverty and a lack of intelligence. But what people often don't understand is a) just how hard it is to be in a bigger body, and b) that there are often many varied and valid reasons – physical, psychological, genetic and socio-economic – *why* people are in bigger bodies in the first place.

The truth is that being fat isn't always a choice. And it's *incredibly* hard. If you asked them, I'm pretty sure most people in bigger bodies would say they'd like to be smaller, if for no other reason than they'd like to be judged less.

A 2016 study by Flint et al. (Flint is Associate Professor of the Psychology of Obesity at the University of Leeds, England) found that overweight and obese[*] individuals were less likely to be offered a job after an interview than thinner applicants. This was true even when the overweight and obese applicants had higher levels of qualifications and job performance. And a 2012 study by US researchers Fikkan and Rothblum found that overweight and obese individuals were less likely

---

[*] I have included these terms as per the language of the study, but we will explore why they're problematic in later chapters ...

to be hired as managers, and were perceived as less competent and less committed than their thinner counterparts.

It's no surprise, then, that the stigma fat people face has a direct impact on both their physical and mental health, and has even been linked to higher levels of anxiety, depression, poor self-esteem and even suicidal ideation. Dr Joshua Wolrich, an NHS doctor, nutritionist and the author of *Food Isn't Medicine*, says weight *stigma* has the potential to have a greater impact on a person's health than their actual weight, which fascinates me.

A lot of people think being fat is a moral failing: a cardinal sin that we choose to commit because we are slovenly, stupid or lacking in willpower. And if you try to explain just how hard it is being in a bigger body, they will often present you with the throw-away, simplistic suggestion of "Just lose weight, then", or, maybe worse, "Have you tried keto?"

It's like they think the idea of trying to lose weight has never even crossed our minds. Whereas, in reality, most of us (myself included, as you've already heard) have been there, done that, bought the T-shirt (several times) and just put the weight all back on (and more).

The truth is: not everyone can lose weight. Nor does everyone want to.

Saying "just lose weight" is a huge oversimplification. It sets the expectation that fat people must embark on a painful, never-ending quest for thinness. And it makes it seem like that would be the answer to everything, rather than there being an urgent need to reshape our ideas about fatness not being inherently bad in the first place. (We'll come on to the idea of weight and health in Chapter 6.)

It also ignores the fact that no diet or exercise programme has ever been proven fully effective for widespread, sustainable, long-term weight loss. In fact, there's a statistic that gets bandied about that claims 95% of diets fail, based on the notion that even if weight loss is achieved at the beginning, this mostly doesn't last.

According to the *American Journal of Public Health*, women who are categorised as "obese" in terms of BMI (30 or over) have an extraordinarily low chance of ever reaching a "healthy" BMI in their lifetime. So, while people are often well-meaning when they say things like "just lose weight", it can feel like they are conveying their superiority – and your failure. "What, like it's hard?" Well, yes, actually, it is.

In addition, it ignores the fact that, for many people, weight loss is intrinsically linked to the way they feel about themselves – often their mental health – so saying "just lose weight" without addressing what's going on in our brains is, to be honest, ridiculous. It's akin to telling someone with depression to "just cheer up".

For too long now, too much focus has been placed on *weight* when it comes to measuring health, when health is, in fact, much more multi-faceted than that. And, ultimately, it's good *health* that should be our goal – not how much gravity we exert on the Earth (more on this in Chapter 6).

IMPLICIT, OR UNCONSCIOUS, BIAS

Some people just hate fat people. And they own that. And they're assholes. This kind of intentional, deliberate prejudice is called explicit bias.

But countless other people aren't even aware that they hold inbuilt biases against fat people, and might be shocked if someone pointed out to them that their words or actions were prejudicial. This is called implicit, or unconscious, bias.

Implicit bias is a term that describes the associations we hold outside of our awareness and control. Think of them as sort of unintentional, knee-jerk reactions. We all have them and, more often than not, they're influenced by our upbringing and personal experiences, as well as by societal stereotypes.

Both types of bias can be harmful. If a doctor were to display explicit anti-fat bias by refusing to treat a patient because of their weight, for example, it could have serious consequences for a person's health and wellbeing. And if another doctor were to display implicit, or unconscious, bias by assuming that a patient's health issues were related to their weight without thoroughly evaluating their medical history and symptoms (a bias that can stem from stereotypes and assumptions about larger-bodied individuals being unhealthy or lacking self-control), it could result in inadequate medical care, as the doctor may overlook critical symptoms or prescribe inappropriate treatments.

Acknowledging our biases is a matter of recognising the social contexts that encourage them. My own biases, for example, will be based on the fact I grew up as a female in a predominantly white, working-class suburban town in England.

As someone who advocates for fat people on a daily basis, I was mortified when I had to complete unconscious bias training at work a few years ago, and my test results revealed I had a very high bias *against* fat people. It showed, like the research mentioned above, I was less likely to hire someone that was in a bigger body, and less likely to see that person as trustworthy.

I wondered for a long time whether this was because I had experienced anti-fat bias throughout my life. But studies show it's a much wider, more ingrained problem than that. A study released by Harvard University in 2019 analysed 4.4 million tests of implicit and explicit bias to examine changes over time in people's attitudes about body weight – along with their feelings about sexual orientation, race, skin tone, age and disability. And the results are uncomfortable to read …

In the course of a decade, the researchers discovered that attitudes about most of these social groups improved (with the majority moving towards neutrality). But while explicit bias towards people who are "overweight" had decreased – and all the other implicit biases studied had either improved or remained stable – *implicit* weight bias had *increased* by 40% between roughly 2004 and 2010.

Data from the *National Survey of Midlife Development in the United States* (MIDUS) even shows that the prevalence of weight discrimination has increased by 66% over the past decade, and is now comparable to prevalence rates of racial discrimination, especially among women. And this rise in unconscious bias has a knock-on effect for women in more ways than one:

Women earn less as they gain weight
A 2015 paper from Vanderbilt University Law School, in Tennessee, found that women categorised as obese were more likely to work in lower-paying, physically demanding jobs, such as elder care or food prep. Another survey, in which the attitudes of more than 500 hiring managers towards potential employers were tested, 21% described the largest woman there as "lazy and unprofessional", only 18% said she had leadership potential and, worse still, only 15% said they would consider hiring her.

It gets worse. Even if fat women get a job, they're likely to be paid less than their smaller counterparts. Scientists at the University of Exeter, in England, found that women who were just 1 stone (14 lb/6 kg) over their "ideal" weight according to the BMI scale, earned around £1,500 ($1,900) a year less than thinner women.

In the US, there are even bigger salary inequities. A 2011 study published by the *Journal of Applied Psychology* found "very thin" women earned $22,000 more than women who were an average size. What's more, fat women earned $9,000 less than their average-sized counterparts. All quite shocking, isn't it?

Fat women get inferior medical care

Hands up if you've ever been to see your doctor and been told to lose weight, despite the problem you went in for being completely unrelated?

Sadly, a lot of doctors are more likely to decide that your issue may be solved if you try harder to lose weight, and, as mentioned a few paragraphs ago, this is sometimes at the expense of doing the tests to properly diagnose you. I've spoken to hundreds of women in recent years whose ailments, including cancer, have gone undiagnosed because doctors refused to take them seriously. I've spoken to hundreds more who say they simply won't visit their doctor any more for fear of being weighed, being told to lose weight or being fat-shamed (whether deliberately or not). See Chapter 6 to hear more about the experiences of a number of such women.

While there are some fantastic healthcare professionals in the medical community who are working to combat fatphobia, they – as members of our weight-obsessed society – are, of course, also subject to its biases.

There's more on fatphobia and health in Chapter 6, but for now here's a little public service announcement: you *can* refuse to be weighed at the doctors if you want. There are even little cards you can print off to show the doctor; these tell them you have a history of eating disorders and/or disordered eating and do not want to be weighed or have your weight discussed unless it is medically necessary (such as for issuing the correct dosage of medication).

Fat-shaming causes stress, depression, anxiety and even eating disorders

The harm, both physical and mental, that fat-shaming can cause is well documented. Studies show that exposure to weight bias can trigger physiological and behavioural changes linked to poor metabolic health and increased weight gain. "You actually experience a form of stress," says Angela Alberga, an assistant professor in the Department of Health, Kinesiology and Applied Physiology at Concordia University in Canada. "Cortisol spikes, self-control drops and the risk of binge-eating increases."

According to Alberga, the more people are exposed to weight bias and discrimination, the more likely they are to gain weight and become fat, even if they were thin to begin with. They're also more likely to die from any cause, regardless of their BMI (body mass index).

And it's not just fat people who are affected, either. Many people with anorexia report that being the victim of fat-shaming on social media contributed to the development of their eating disorder. They say that once they began losing weight by not eating, exercising obsessively and abusing laxatives or diuretics, the positive feedback they received (including on social media) further encouraged them to intensify their behaviour.

THE DEVASTATING IMPACT OF WEIGHT STIGMA

We know by now that the world certainly isn't always kind to you when you're in a bigger body, or any type of marginalised body, for that matter.

I always find it funny that you tend to be both invisible and *hyper* visible when you're fat. In public, you're a walking target: something to be gawped at (or, even worse, laughed at). But in the wider sense of the world, your worth and your weight are often so intrinsically linked that the bigger you are, the less your value in society is.

People who have never experienced weight stigma will never know the fear we feel when faced with public transport, drunk men or a group of chatty children (or those awful, tiny white plastic chairs that seem to make an appearance at every family BBQ).

The world is simply not accommodating to, or designed for, bigger bodies. And I'm not even talking about *very* large bodies.

Take aeroplanes, for example. Anyone above a UK size 16 (the national average, and the equivalent of a US size 12) struggles to fit into a seat comfortably and may need a seatbelt extender. While statistics show that, as a society, we've all gotten fatter, standard plane seats have actually shrunk. They're now just 17 inches (43 cm) instead of 18.5 inches (47 cm). And leg room has also shrunk from 35 inches (89 cm) to 31 inches (79 cm) in the last decade. For lots of us, the bliss of going on holiday is therefore often weighed down by the stress and discomfort of air travel.

Flying is actually one of my biggest fears. This is partly because I'm an anxious person who thinks we're going to crash and die at the slightest hint of any turbulence (my poor husband), but mainly it's because I know it's many people's worse nightmare to be sat next to someone who looks like me. You only need to scan Twitter to see how disgusted and angry people can get when they have to sit next to someone who is on the larger side. Often, images are taken of passengers without their consent or knowledge – just for them to be ridiculed in the most humiliating, public way.

"A disgust that otherwise lies dormant reveals itself in airplanes," says fat activist Gordon. And she's right. I recently came back from a holiday that required a long-haul flight and a short(ish) flight on a seaplane. For weeks leading up to the holiday, I worried about fitting in the seat, having to ask for a seatbelt extender, who I would be sat next to, what I should wear to look "less fat", whether to apologise to the person next to me or not, whether I would be weighed before getting on the seaplane, whether I would fit on the seaplane, if they would have an extender, if people would complain they felt unsafe with me on board, how easily I would be able to walk through the aisle, how quickly I'd be able to get on and off, the judgemental looks …

On this occasion, it was actually OK. The seatbelt on the seaplane was (surprisingly) almost twice the length of those on a standard plane, and, although it was hot and a bit crammed, I almost, almost, enjoyed it.

But this has not always been the case. I've had a few bad experiences on flights over the years. About 10 years ago, shortly after boarding a plane to Germany for a work trip, I realised my seatbelt didn't do up, and my body swelled with heat and embarrassment. I wasn't prepared for it. At all.

I tried to pretend it did by strategically hovering my arm over it, but the flight attendant clocked me and told me I needed a seatbelt extender. The 21-year-old me was mortified as she paraded this bright orange thing through the aisle and waved it in my face. It was made worse by two teenage girls nearby, who found my humiliation to be a source of entertainment. I had to endure giggling, laughing, pointing and them taking pictures of me throughout the entire flight – and it was mortifying.

With age comes confidence, though, and, while I still have my wobbles, I'm now a lot happier flying than I was. I used to bring my own seatbelt with me, and always wore a scarf no matter how hot it was to hide said seatbelt. Now, I wear whatever I'm comfortable in and I ask for an extender as soon as I get on the plane. (See also Chapter 8 for more on the experience of flying as a bigger-bodied person, including a box of top tips on flying when fat.)

It isn't always easy, but the alternative is sitting at home and missing out on opportunities to travel and make memories. And that's not a life I want for me, or for you. I try to remind myself that holidays are a privilege.

My biggest wish is that we, as a society, start to acknowledge how rife anti-fat bias is and put the onus more on dismantling it (and being more accommodating to individuals) than trying to "fix" people. Because it's not just our physical health that suffers, but our mental health too.

In a 2010 study published in the journal *Obesity*, researchers found that weight stigma was associated with higher levels of depression and lower levels of life satisfaction among women with obesity. "Our findings highlight the importance of addressing weight stigma as a public health issue, and not just a personal problem," said lead author Andrea Garber, PhD, RD, of the University of California, San Francisco.

Weight stigma can also have a negative impact on eating behaviours and body image. A 2019 study published in the *International Journal of Eating Disorders* found that women who experienced weight stigma were more likely to engage in emotional eating and had higher levels of body dissatisfaction.

RECLAIMING THE "F" WORD

Hopefully, by now you've started to realise – if you didn't already know – just how rife anti-fat bias is in our society, and that unconscious bias is something we all have to work harder to fight against, whatever our size.

As we reach the end of this chapter, let's talk about how important it is that we reclaim the word "fat".

"Fat" is a word that many people avoid, and understandably so, as many of us have spent a lifetime being conditioned to think of it as deeply cruel. As we touched on earlier, the idea of being fat has often had negative connotations, such as laziness, lack of self-control, unattractiveness and even moral failure. This cultural stigma has led to many people avoiding using it altogether – or using other words instead, like "curvy", "voluptuous", "full-figured" or "plus size".

I understand that use of the word, or not, is a personal choice, but I also think that it's imperative we reclaim the word fat as a neutral descriptor, similar to other physical characteristics like "tall," "short" or "brunette". Because using euphemisms, or avoiding the word altogether, only reinforces the sense of shame and stigma associated with being fat, and the idea that it's not possible to be fat and healthy, fat and beautiful, fat and successful, etc.

Of course, not everyone is comfortable being called fat. Even for me personally, it's challenging, given that the word was a source of such pain and fear for such a long time. I have no issue with calling *myself* fat. Because I am. But I'd be lying if I said I was completely comfortable with other people calling me it, especially as almost every minor altercation I've ever had has always started or ended with being called a "fat b****" or a "fat c***".

But I think, for things to change, we all need to get more comfortable with the idea of reclaiming the word and using it.

Fat activist Gordon says: "It requires challenging deeply ingrained beliefs and attitudes, both within ourselves and within our society. It requires acknowledging the pain and trauma that fatphobia has caused, while also refusing to be defined by it. It requires a commitment to self-love and self-acceptance, even in the face of societal pressure to conform to narrow beauty standards."

When it comes to denying that someone else is fat in an effort to placate them, Gordon says that it actually overlooks a significant aspect of their lived experience and ignores the biases and discrimination they face. So, when a fat person calls themselves fat (as a straightforward recognition that they're not thin), we need to respect that, because it's their personal choice to call themselves that. Although this changes, of course, if they're using the term in a derogatory way about *themselves*, such as by saying something like "I'm fat and ugly", in which case reminding them to be kinder to themselves is perfectly OK.

"Being called fat isn't just about a changing body, it's about subjugation to a culture that marginalises and stigmatises fat individuals," says Gordon. "But for fat folk, reclaiming the word fat is about reclaiming our bodies and our right to name them."

SELF-EMPOWERMENT TASK

Take a little time out for yourself and ask yourself how you feel about the word "fat".

What emotions and/or memories does it bring up for you? Do you feel comfortable using the word in a neutral way, whether about yourself or others? And do you think you hold any bias, whether conscious or unconscious, towards people who are in a bigger body than yours?

Feel free to write down anything that feels particularly powerful in case it might help you to get any negative thoughts and feelings on this topic out of your system.

3

"F*** your beauty standards"

The fickle world of the beauty industry

I can't say I paid much attention to what I looked like when I was very young. My mum was always trying to get me to wear pretty pink dresses, but every day I wasn't at school, I would head straight to my brother's wardrobe and pick out one of his T-shirts and a pair of cargo shorts. I remember one dress in particular that had buttons down the back and a white collar. Every time it was waved in my face (normally alongside a bribe to wear it), I would throw a tantrum. *"I'm not wearing that and you can't make me!"*

On rare occasions I might let my mum brush my hair and put it in a ponytail, but for the most part I wasn't interested in how I looked, and because of this I was labelled a "tomboy". I think for a long time I just wanted to be like my brother. Not only because I looked up to him, but also because of how simple it was for him to just "be". I learned from a young age that boys were supposed to be (and allowed to be) strong, fast and adventurous. And girls were just supposed to be "pretty". But I wasn't interested in looking pretty. I wanted to be one of the boys. I believed I would never look like the girls and celebrities featured on those pages, so I took myself out of the race, so to speak, and instead started eating more to comfort myself.

That all changed, however, when I started reading magazines like *Mizz* and *Seventeen*. Hidden among the glossy pages full of beauty advice and dating tips were insidious messages about how we should look and behave and, funnily enough, the products we should buy in order to obtain that image.

In an attempt to gain a sense of validation and self-worth, I felt an overwhelming need to overcompensate for my perceived physical shortcomings by trying to be hyper feminine. I would wear pretty, "flattering" dresses, apply my makeup meticulously, and keep my hair long and perfectly styled.

Those magazines, along with the lack of representation and blatant fat-shaming on TV, left me feeling pretty worthless. I didn't fit Western society's beauty standards, and that meant I felt lesser than (despite being bigger than) all of my friends.

It wasn't until I was about 25 that I started questioning what I saw in magazines and in the media. Seeing Kim Kardashian on the cover of *Papier* magazine was a real turning point. You can probably picture it: she posed in a revealing black dress while balancing a champagne glass on her newly inflated ass. For me, this was the start of us seeing not just unrealistic beauty standards, but impossible ones.

After the magazine cover dropped, lots of people raced to get surgical procedures, or they bought bum-sculpting leggings or started a new fad workout that targeted the glutes. Then, less than five years later, small bums were back in fashion and everyone was asking "Does my bum look big in this?" again.

It made me realise just how pathetic these ever-changing, unrealistic beauty standards are, and how truly fucked up it is that we, as women, are supposed to conform to them.

And it's not just our bodies, either; it's our hair, our make-up, our body hair, our skin ... We've never really stood a chance to be "allowed" to love ourselves, have we? In this chapter we're going to look at body ideals through the years and explore how unrealistic beauty standards wreak havoc with our self-esteem. It's time to give such unrealistic standards the middle finger they deserve.

A HISTORY OF CHANGING BODY TRENDS

Body trends aren't a new phenomenon. And here's a fun fact for you: thin hasn't always been "in", even as far back as ancient Greece. In that time, Aphrodite was known as a beautiful and alluring goddess of love, beauty and fertility, with artistic representations emphasising her curves and voluptuousness. And when we look at the Renaissance period in Europe (from the 14th to 17th centuries), bigger women were seen as powerful and beautiful. Some even saw being skinny as unattractive. You only have to google "Renaissance art" to see a plethora of fuller-figured beauties, including the Mona Lisa. If you're wondering why, it's because being heavier showed that you not only had money, but that you also had key signs of fertility (i.e. larger breasts and bigger hips), making you a more desirable prospect for marriage.

This trend for a more curvaceous figure continued well into the Victorian era with the introduction of corsets, designed to create the illusion of an hourglass figure. In 1867, a regular series appeared in the fashion magazine *Harper's Bazaar* called "For the Ugly Girls", which told women they needed to be "comelier and rounder" than the "scrawny, sallow peaked woman" of the past, but not "become gross and obese, as so many of their European sisters".

Even back then women were being told of the parameters within which their body would be deemed acceptable. Curvy, but not too curvy. Busty, but not too busty. Slim, but not too slim. Sound familiar?

Harper's Bazaar went on to carry the mantle for the "right" models of beauty for women for decades after that, all of which were based on both class and race. It even denounced the fatness of the "savage races" and said women of colour could only be deemed attractive if they adhered to Western ideals of beauty, i.e. narrow nose, coral lips, white teeth, small mouth.

It wasn't until the 1920s, when fashion and society increasingly placed a greater emphasis on the role of women in society, that the desire for a slimmer, more androgynous look became desirable. The 1920s was an exciting time for women's rights, with many new opportunities and roles arising in the wake of women having taken on traditionally male roles during the war effort of the previous decade. But, despite this, women were still expected to conform to the beauty ideals of the time and, just like today, this expectation placed an immense amount of pressure on them – affecting not only their own self-image, but also their public standing.

Thanks to the 20th-century emergence of mass advertising and the rising power of the fashion industry, it was strongly hinted to women that they needed to be slim and attractive – or risk being ostracised from society. Fashion magazines depicted boyish figures with small hips, small breasts and a defined waist as the epitome of beauty. And extreme diets were published left, right and centre, which meant there was suddenly a pressure and expectation on women to not only be the perfect housewife, but to be thin to boot. The traditional hourglass corset was replaced by a rubber girdle to retract the hips, and the emergence of mass-produced clothing led to the creation of assigned body sizes for women and a defined body type. Clothes were no longer made to fit a person's body. Instead, the person's body had to conform to the clothes.

There were even adverts that suggested it was a woman's "duty" to maintain her appearance in order for her husband not to stray. It really is a wonder how a man's inability to keep his dick in his pants can be blamed on his wife not being "comely" enough or having the right haircut! I despair.

WOMEN'S BODIES SHOULD NOT BE TRENDS

Since the 1920s, when super thin was all the rage, the ideal body type has continued to shift – from voluptuous to androgynous to muscular, and everything in between. And as these ideals change, they are reflected and reinforced in the culture through media – whether it's fine art, fashion magazines, billboards or music videos.

In the past three decades, the celebrated body has also veered wildly, from large-breasted to small, big-bummed to little, and large-lipped to neat-mouthed. The trend for lip fillers has been growing stronger by the day, yet at the same time some people view them as tacky, which means that those who dissolve their fillers and post videos about embracing their natural beauty are met with high praise online. Girls with enhanced lips are seen as on trend, but they also risk seeming insecure – someone without the inner confidence we're now all suddenly supposed to have.

It really does feel like women can't win.

And let's not forget the way female beauty standards vary between cultures. In Mauritania, young girls are brutally force-fed a diet of up to 16,000 calories a day to get them big enough for marriage. For the Māori people of New Zealand, nothing says beauty like a tattoo on your face – which is traditionally done with a chisel (ouch).

In Western society, a recent trend for big bums saw women getting (and dying from) Brazilian Butt Lifts (BBLs) – a surgical procedure that involves transferring fat from another part of the body to the buttocks. This has been identified as one of the most dangerous cosmetic procedures, with a mortality rate of one in 3,000 cases, significantly higher than other common cosmetic surgeries, such as breast augmentation, which has a mortality rate of one in 50,000 cases. Yet, now, it seems that the trend for big bums is on its way out already!

Viewed as a whole, beauty culture starts to look nothing short of abusive. It asks us to harm ourselves for its pleasure; then changes its mind and wants us to harm ourselves differently. It pressures us to appear a certain way, then mocks us for trying so hard to please. It demands impossible things.

In 2020, actress and singer Cynthia Erivo delivered a powerful speech about beauty standards at the *Essence* Black Women in Hollywood Awards. She spoke about how society's beauty standards have often excluded women of colour and how she had to overcome feelings of insecurity and inadequacy in order to embrace her own natural beauty. "We have been taught to hate ourselves for things that are not even within our control, and it's time for that to end," she said. "We have to start telling ourselves a different story about who we are and what we look like. We have to start celebrating our own unique beauty."

After all these years, we should consider the possibility that female insecurity is not, in fact, an unfortunate side effect of beauty culture, but a very deliberate end goal. Perhaps starved, anxious and humiliated women are much easier to push around – and sell stuff to!

It seems to me that, perhaps, in a patriarchal society that was made "for men, by men", impossible female standards have been created to wear women down, both physically and psychologically, which makes them easier to control.

BODY IDEALS OVER THE PAST 100 YEARS

Throughout the 20th and 21st centuries, the idea of the "perfect body shape" for women (i.e. how women "should" look!) has shifted continuously. So let's take a quick jaunt through the decades – so I can prove to you what a load of bollocks body trends are.

1910s: The Gibson Girl
The Gibson Girl was the ideal feminine body type of the 1910s. The look was tall and slender, with a small waist and a "boyish" body shape. Women at the time strived to achieve this look by wearing corsets that cinched their waists, giving them a looping figure-8 shape. This silhouette was popularised through illustrations by Charles Gibson and appearances in magazines such as *LIFE*, *Collier's* and *Harper's Bazaar*. Women who embodied the Gibson Girl look were seen as independent and modern, a sharp contrast to the look of the Victorian era that preceded it.

1920s: The Flapper Girl
Curves were out and a smaller bust and hips were in. This look was streamlined and petite, and the focus moved to women's legs, as shorter hemlines of flapper dresses put them on display. Women also embraced

a more boyish figure, often wearing bandeau bras to flatten their chests. The androgynous look was further emphasised by the fashion trends of the era, with short haircuts and minimal makeup.

1930s: The fitted silhouette

In the 1930s, a more fitted silhouette was in fashion, with a slight return to a curvaceous figure. The waistline moved several inches below the navel, requiring narrow hips, and the focus of femininity shifted even more to the legs, with now shorter hemlines exposing the flash of a garter while dancing the shimmy. Margaret Gorman, the first Miss America in 1921, was seen as the embodiment of this ideal, with her 5ft 1in (150 cm), 7.7 stone (108 lb/49 kg) frame. The look was elegant, with an emphasis on understated glamour.

1940s: The angular body

During World War II, women's expanding roles in the workforce influenced fashion, leading to an angular body type becoming the ideal. The look was commanding, with broad, boxy shoulders and a tall, square silhouette. Women's clothing reflected their newfound responsibilities, with utility clothing such as pants and jumpsuits becoming more popular.

1950s: The hourglass figure

Marilyn Monroe paved the way for a more voluptuous and curvy body type in the 1950s, with a small waist and large bust. The creation of *Playboy* magazine and Barbie also had a big part to play in influencing the fashions of the time. Sweetheart necklines and circle skirts were all the rage, in an attempt to highlight the ideal hourglass shape. Women were encouraged to embrace their femininity and curves, with shapewear like bullet bras and girdles being popular.

1960s: The androgynous figure

The swinging '60s saw a move back towards a slim and androgynously trim figure, with a focus on a flat stomach and small bust and hips. Models such as Twiggy and Jean Shrimpton graced every catwalk and magazine cover, embodying the mod look of the time. Weight Watchers launched in New York in 1963, catapulting a cultural pressure to maintain a slim figure through diet.

1970s: Disco

In the 1970s, jumpsuits and big hair were all the rage. The slim body type continued to be popular, but with a more natural and relaxed appearance. There was also a rise in the popularity of fitness and healthy living, with a greater acceptance of a range of body types. Women's liberation movements also had an impact on fashion, with clothing becoming more unisex and practical.

1980s: The Amazonian supermodel

The 1980s marked a significant shift in the fashion industry, with the emergence of the Amazonian supermodels. Elle MacPherson and Naomi Campbell were among the tall, leggy women who became the new feminine ideal. The supermodels dominated not just the runway, but also print and television ads. With their striking features, they represented a departure from the traditional model look of the past. Another trend that emerged in the 1980s was fitness, thanks to the one and only Jane Fonda. Her fitness videos inspired a generation of people to embrace exercise and healthy living. Aerobics and jogging became popular and, for the first time, muscles were considered "in" for both men and women.

1990s: Heroin chic

Supermodel Kate Moss ushered in a new era of fashion in the 1990s with her waifish look. The gaunt appearance, which is now popularly known as "heroin chic", became a trend, alongside slouchy jeans, oversized, fraying sweaters, and bomber jackets. It was a stark contrast to the previous decade's Amazonian supermodels, with their toned bodies and striking features. In 1996, The New York Times referred to '90s fashion as "a pusher of what appears to be the best-dressed heroin addicts in history". The waif look also represented a significant cultural shift towards a more grunge and alternative aesthetic, which influenced fashion and music.

2000s: Athletic

Gisele Bündchen marked the end of the era of "heroin chic" in the early 2000s. With her toned stomach and long legs, she became the epitome of the new feminine ideal. The pale, gaunt, glass-eyed look of the '90s was replaced by visible abs and airbrushed tans. Bündchen was crowned "The Most Beautiful Girl in the World" by *Rolling Stone* magazine and became a dominating force in the fashion industry, from print ads to Victoria's Secret lingerie shows. Her healthy and athletic look represented a shift towards a more natural, toned beauty standard.

2010s: Bootylicious

Nicki Minaj and Jennifer Lopez became the poster girls for the almighty buttock in this decade, inspiring a new trend in fashion and beauty. Kim Kardashian famously "broke the internet" with her backside, which sparked a sharp rise in people going under the knife for the trendy but dangerous Brazilian Butt Lift procedure mentioned earlier. The fitness industry also embraced the trend, with new workouts designed to target the glutes.

2020s: The return of "heroin chic"

The 2020s have marked a resurgence of '90s fashion trends, including the return of "heroin chic", with models in fashion campaigns and runway shows sporting the same gaunt, skeletal look that was popular then. Brands like Saint Laurent, Balenciaga and Calvin Klein received criticism for featuring models with dangerously low body weights, which sparked concern among health advocates and eating disorder experts. The debate surrounding body image and the fashion industry continues to be contentious, with the need for diversity and inclusivity at the forefront of the conversation.

WHY ARE WOMEN'S BODIES NOT ALLOWED TO AGE?

Our society is not only obsessed with thinness, but also the pursuit of eternal youth.

The natural process of ageing is often weaponised against women, with anti-ageing creams and lotions promising to "turn back time" being advertised and sold by the millions every year. We're also made to feel as if we've failed if we don't have a body like J.Lo at age 54, when, in reality, she's the exception, not the rule.

There's no getting away from the fact that, as we age, our bodies change. Skin loses elasticity, wrinkles form and muscles weaken. Yet society's expectations of female beauty remain rigid and unforgiving, with ageing and sagging skin often seen as flaws to be fixed or hidden.

"Women are bombarded with messages that ageing is something to be feared and that their value is tied to their youthful appearance," says Dr Renee Engeln, author of *Beauty Sick: How the Cultural Obsession with Appearance Hurts Girls and Women*. "This creates a constant pressure to maintain a certain standard of beauty that is unrealistic and impossible to achieve."

The effects of these messages are far-reaching. A study published in the *Journal of Women & Aging* in 2008 found that negative attitudes towards ageing were associated with lower levels of self-esteem and life satisfaction in middle-aged women. Another study published in the same journal in 2019 found that women who experienced body dissatisfaction were more likely to develop depression and anxiety.

These messages are also perpetuated in media and advertising. Images of young, flawless models are pervasive, creating a standard that is unattainable for most women, which can lead to a feeling of constant inadequacy.

The global anti-ageing market is predicted to grow from $191.5 billion in 2019 to a whopping $421.4 billion by 2030, according to market research company P&S Intelligence. However, despite Gen X women (born from the mid-1960s to the mid-1980s) outspending both Baby Boomers (born in the years after the Second World War) and Millennials (born in the 1980s and 1990s), few publications and brands actually market to these women or use them in their advertising. Have you noticed the vast majority of adverts feature models who are in their early 30s or 40s (and who are also normally light-skinned, white and heavily edited)? It's no wonder, then, that a lot of older women say they are made to feel invisible by the lack of representation.

What's really gross is that brands know this, and literally make them pay the price for it. Anti-ageing products are known to be some of the most expensive in the skincare market. In a 2010 investigation by UK newspaper *The Daily Mail*, it was found that recreating a 100g pot (3.4 oz) of the highly popular Crème de la Mer from readily available ingredients cost around £9.71 ($12) to make. That's about £14.50 ($17) in today's money. Pretty cheap when you compare it to the current £435 ($540) price tag.

As women, we are constantly subject to consumer culture treating our bodies as capital. And this can have a big impact on the way we view ourselves. In our culture, ageing is often viewed as a loss of value, as we associate it with the loss of our beauty (deemed by the patriarchy as our biggest asset).

The impact of ageism on self-esteem is compounded when we consider the differences in how the process of growing older is perceived between men and women. Have you noticed how men are never targeted by the anti-ageing market? Or at least, not to the same degree. This normalised idea that men are allowed to age while women must always look young is reinforced in various ways, such as the continuous casting of younger women as the love interests of older men in Hollywood films.

The beauty industry also perpetuates this perception through language, often using negative connotations like "decline" and "ageing" to describe the process of women getting older.

Grey hair was widely accepted as normal until 1940, when an ad by Clairol suggested greys were responsible for a woman's dwindling social life. The ad read "Are your friends drifting away from you ... finding excuses to break appointments ... failing to call you? That happens so very often to a grey-haired woman ... sometimes because people think she looks too old to have fun ... sometimes because they think she looks too old to *be* fun." And, pretty much ever since, women with grey hair have been encouraged to dye it, while phrases like "silver fox" are used to glorify older men with greying hair.

Wrinkles on women are also often viewed as making them look old, tired, unhealthy or "past it". In contrast, men with wrinkles are often talked of as ageing like a "fine wine". The phrase "ageing gracefully" is used all the time to commend someone for not displaying any signs of the natural process, particularly wrinkles. This further reinforces the idea that ageing is something to be ashamed of, particularly for women.

In Hollywood, facelifts are still practically demanded of older actresses, but beware the "insecure victims" who get them done. Tabloids will either say something like, "She's looking remarkably fresh-faced", or, as was the case with Madonna recently, "What on Earth has she done to her face?"

I realise this chapter has been a bit doom and gloom so far, so I want to point out there are signs the beauty industry is changing and beginning to realise the importance of using language and imagery that accurately reflects people's diverse experiences of ageing.

The Body Shop's recent decision to rename its best-selling "Drops of Youth" serum to "Edelweiss" was a small win. And Dove now also advocates for allowing women to "age beautifully on their own terms". Its #KeepTheGrey campaign takes a stand against ageist expectations and double standards in the workplace for women with grey hair.

This empowering campaign was launched in response to the outcry surrounding the replacement of Lisa LaFlamme – a long-standing, award-winning news broadcaster on Canadian TV (CTV) – with a younger male. Executives at CTV, where LaFlamme had worked for 35 years, had reportedly asked who had approved the news anchor's decision to let her hair go grey. A storm then erupted on social media about ageism and sexism in the media, and this is where Dove stepped in. The campaign was widely praised for promoting inclusivity and diversity in the beauty industry. Let's hope it's the start of many to come.

EUROCENTRIC BEAUTY STANDARDS

It's not just older women the beauty industry has hurt. Women of colour have been, and still are, consistently excluded from the mainstream thanks to Eurocentric ideals.

Eurocentric beauty standards are those that prioritise features commonly associated with European traits, such as fair skin, narrow noses, thin lips and straight hair. These standards have been perpetuated by Western media and often exclude people of colour who do not fit within these constricted definitions of beauty.

For decades, Eurocentric beauty standards have been the norm in the fashion industry and media. With tall, thin, predominantly white models gracing the covers of magazines and runways, these standards have reinforced a limited and exclusive definition of beauty that has left many feeling excluded and inadequate. While they might seem like something that is relegated to the cover of a magazine, they permeate society – from places of work and education to social dynamics and internal worth.

"The problem with Eurocentric beauty standards is that they are not inclusive of the vast diversity that exists in the world," says Dr Sarah E Gaither, Associate Professor of Psychology and Neuroscience at Duke University. "By privileging certain physical characteristics, we are essentially saying that certain people are more valued than others."

These ideals have harmful effects on people's mental health and self-esteem. A study published in the *Journal of Black Psychology* found that black women who internalised Eurocentric beauty ideals had lower self-esteem and were more likely to develop eating disorders.

Furthermore, these ideals also have implications for representation in the media and fashion industry. "When the only standard of beauty is Eurocentric, it excludes people of different races, ethnicities, and body types," says Gaither. "It's important to recognise and embrace the diversity that exists in our world."

The origins of Eurocentric beauty standards can be traced back to colonialism and the concept of white superiority. During this time, Europeans travelled to other parts of the world and imposed their cultural beliefs and standards on the people they encountered. This included the idea that light skin was a sign of status and beauty, while darker skin was associated with being lower class.

One of the most significant ways Eurocentric beauty standards have manifested is through the focus on light skin. In many cultures, fair skin is considered a desirable trait, and skin-lightening products are widely used. In some cases, these products can be really harmful, leading to skin damage and even cancer.

A skin-lightening cream called "Fair & Lovely", patented by Hindustan Unilever and marketed towards women since 1975, became one of the biggest cosmetic products in South Asia. Its immense popularity goes to show just how ingrained the notion is in South Asian cultures that dark skin can't be lovely. It was only in 2020, due to a great uproar against its colourist connotations, that "Fair & Lovely" was renamed "Glow & Lovely".

Going back in time, the ancient Greeks also used to lust for pale skin. In fact, throughout history it was considered a luxury because it indicated that a woman didn't have to spend her days outside, working in the sun. Such was the perceived status of light skin that Italian Renaissance women adopted the use of "ceruse" (a white carbonate of lead, ground up into a powder), and mixed this with vinegar for a full-face application; from there, they painted on raw egg white to achieve a glowing, dewy complexion. Similarly, in Elizabethan times, women, including Queen Elizabeth I herself, would lighten their faces with white lead and sometimes even chalk.

The association between beauty and whiteness has proven hard to shake, and there's a reason so many people still think of an "all-American beauty" as a thin, blonde, blue-eyed white woman. It wasn't until 1940 that the rules were changed to allow women of colour to enter the Miss America pageant. Before that, the official rules stated contestants had to be "of good health and of the white race".

I recently asked six women of colour about their experience with conforming to Eurocentric beauty standards. Here are their stories:

When I was in secondary school, I was one of two black people. I never wore my hair down as my mum and dad didn't know what to do with it. I desperately wanted long, straight hair like everyone else. I tried a chemical relaxer four times as a teenager, but all it did was leave me with considerable hair loss. My body changed a lot during this time too, and I developed big boobs and thick thighs. People commented a lot on my shape, especially my "big African bum", and it was really painful.

I couldn't even find make-up for my skin tone. I wrote to Boots once and told them the make-up they stocked wasn't reflective of the multiculturalism in the UK and they wrote back to say there "wasn't demand for it".
– Becky

Aged 11, I refused to go to secondary school unless my hair was straight. A white hairdresser in my town used European curl chemical straighter on my hair. He thought leaving it on for longer than recommended would work, as my hair was so curly. I was left with bald patches and open wounds. I was also badly bullied about my lips. At school I was told I had DSLs ("dick-sucking lips"), and constantly told they were "too big". Now lip fillers are all the rage, and massive lips are trendy.

When I've spoken out about women who blackfish by getting fillers, people don't understand how something I was bullied for has become an easy off-the-shelf cosmetic procedure.
– Lauren D

I was only about seven when I became aware my skin and hair were different. On the whole now, I don't care as much. But I work in a predominantly white workplace, have to wear a hair covering if I go in the lab, and they're just not designed for people with Afro hair or dreadlocks that are naturally thicker. As a forensic scientist, I also have to go to court sometimes. I'm always aware of my hair and my skin colour, and worry if I'll be taken seriously or professionally. It shouldn't be that way, but it's just something you're always aware of when you're a person of colour.
– Cicely

As an Asian person, it's believed the fairer you are, the more attractive you are (the paler the better against dark hair). So if I ever got a remote hint of a tan, I'd hate it and scrub it for weeks to try and get rid of it. If you look at Bollywood actresses, you even get European women who have learnt Hindi, making a name because they fit the aesthetic better.
– Ammishah

In the US, there has been a history of demonising people of colour for their "exotic" features (narrow eyes, big bum, curly hair, freckles, plush lips, you name it) and then adapting those traits via cosmetic processes, all the while heaping shame on the people to whom those traits come naturally.

When I stopped straightening my hair, I got so many compliments. At first it felt really validating to have something I had always seen as "wrong" be treated as something to value. But, after a while of wearing my hair curly, it started to really grate on me. This was because I started to realise I was getting praise for something that didn't fit with my skin tone (I'm mixed race but with a lighter skin tone) and also for something that the darker women in my family felt was "wrong" about them. My black grandma straightened her hair until she retired, and would refer to her curly hair after she stopped as something she'd "let go", or didn't care enough to change anymore. Something "unprofessional".

Thankfully, now I've reached a sort of neutrality about it, but obviously I still think about it a lot.

– Emma

Being a mixed-race teenager in the noughties was tough! There was no beauty standard apart from straight hair, light skin and skinny. This really did affect my core sense of self growing up. It wasn't till I got older that I realised how badly it had affected me. I turn 30 today, and now I'm super proud of my brown skin, big nose, chubby body and curly hair. It gets better. Sixteen-year-old me would never believe it.

– Lauren R

FEMALE GROOMING AND THE "EW" FACTOR

Did you know that until the early 20th century, both men and women pretty much left their body hair alone?

However, everything changed in the 1900s, when Gillette released its first razor for women, to capitalise on the growth of the female consumer. At the same time, the brand started the first anti-underarm-hair campaign, pushing its product as a necessity.

In 1915, an ad in fashion magazine *Harper's Bazaar* featured a model in a sleeveless dress with her hands above her head. The slogan read: "Summer Dress and Modern Dancing combine to make necessary the removal of objectionable hair."

Until that point, hair removal creams were sold, but their main use was for removing strays on the face and neck. However, after the successful campaign by Gillette, more and more women started to shave their armpits, and it wasn't long before it was considered an essential act of personal hygiene.

Around 20 years later, the same thing happened with leg hair. After the Pearl Harbor attack in 1941, the United States went to war against Japan and, suddenly, the production of nylon was diverted from making stockings to making everything from glider tow ropes and aircraft fuel tanks to flak jackets and parachutes for the military.

After enjoying the benefits of nylon stockings, women didn't want to go back to silk, so they did the next best thing: they shaved their legs, carefully applied a "liquid silk stocking" (otherwise known as paint), and lined the backs of their legs with a trompe l'oeil seam.

This brought in a bold, new revolution that brands capitalised on: leg-hair removal was marketed as replicating the appearance of stockings, and women bought into it hook, line and sinker.

As leg-hair removal grew in popularity, so did the removal of shaving practically any hair that wasn't deemed necessary. The introduction of the bikini in the US in 1946 also led shaving companies and female consumers to focus on trimming down below.

Pre-1980s, the majority of women had sported their natural body hair (hence why the natural look is often known as "1970s bush"). However, as cameras and technology became more advanced, porn videos tended to focus more and more on the intricacies of the vulva. Put simply, where there was less hair, there was more to see. It's thought that this was one of the main catalysts for women shaving their bikini line, or sporting a "landing strip".

It wasn't until more recent years that the Brazilian wax became mainstream. In 1987, seven sisters from Brazil (known as the J Sisters) opened a salon in New York City offering the "Brazilian" – complete hair removal. Celebrities like Gwyneth Paltrow and Naomi Campbell started doing it, and the masses followed suit, with body-hair removal soon becoming the norm.

Fast forward to today, and a new cohort of young women are once again embracing body hair – nowhere more obviously so than on Instagram, although the phenomenon has also made it into magazines. In the September 2019 issue of *Harper's Bazaar*, actress Emily Ratajkowski posed with unshaven underarms, creating a 180-degree turn for the publication since its early anti-armpit-hair messages.

I think more women are realising now how body hair is deeply connected to gender and power. By choosing not to shave or wax, they are using it as a tool for activism and social change, and I'm here for it.

CONFLICTING FEELINGS ABOUT
BEAUTY STANDARDS?

I hear from a lot of women who feel conflicted about wanting to reject beauty standards but still want to be beautiful. And trust me, I get it. Lots of us know female beauty and body standards are bullshit made up by marketers, but still want to wear make-up to feel nice, or revel in getting compliments for dressing up or losing weight.

It's natural to want to reject harmful standards and still desire to meet them. But it's important to remember that trends are unrealistic and unattainable, and that trying to conform to them only creates a sense of inadequacy and self-doubt, as well as an unhealthy preoccupation with appearance. Our bodies are not objects to be perfected, but vehicles that allow us to move through the world and experience life. Wouldn't it be great to celebrate our bodies for all they do for us, rather than trying to force them to conform to unrealistic, or impossible, standards?

However, rejecting body trends doesn't mean we can't take care of ourselves or feel good about our appearance. It simply means recognising there are many different body types and shapes that are beautiful, and we don't have to look a certain way to be worthy of love and respect.

We don't have to have an hourglass figure to be worthy of being seen. Our hair doesn't have to be shiny and silky to make us worthy of being listened to. Our faces don't have to be devoid of wrinkles for us to be worthy of receiving kindness. And we don't have to be cellulite free to be beautiful! (Fun fact: did you know that cellulite wasn't even a thing until 1968, when the US edition of *Vogue* featured a headline on its front page: "Cellulite: the fat you couldn't lose before". In her bestseller book *The Beauty Myth*, feminist journalist Naomi Wolf argues that this resulted in a pop-culture tendency to reinterpret healthy "adult female flesh" as a "condition", which it blatantly is NOT!)

For me, taking back the power means wearing a bit of fake tan every now and again because it makes me feel good, not because I feel I have to. It means experimenting with make-up because I find it fun, not because I feel I have to hide. It means rejecting every new body trend that comes into fashion because I know my body is not, and never will be, a "trend".

SELF-EMPOWERMENT TASK

Take a little time out for yourself and think back to the first time (or times) that you can remember becoming self-conscious about your appearance.

What emotions did it and/or does it bring up for you? And what would you say to your younger self about these experiences now?

Feel free to write down anything that feels particularly triggering and/or powerful to you, in case there are things here that you would like to spend more time working through.

4

The media's obsession with thin

A lack of diversity and a lot of fat stereotypes

Anyone who's ever turned on a television, read a glossy magazine or scrolled through Instagram knows that our society is obsessed with bodies. Specifically, thin bodies. I don't know about you, but I never saw anyone who looked even remotely likely me in magazines or on TV when I was growing up, unless the person was being made fun of. And this had a big effect on me.

As bestselling author and activist Sonya Renee Taylor writes in her book *The Body Is Not an Apology*: "Representation is important because when we don't see ourselves reflected in the world around us, we can't help but make assumptions about that absence. Invisibility is a statement. It says something about the world and our place in it. Difference is equated with undesirability."

In this chapter, we're going to look at the ways in which the media has objectified and scrutinised women's bodies, and, in the process, made us feel shitty about ourselves. They really do have a lot to answer for.

MEDIA EXCLUSION AND MISREPRESENTATION

For the longest time, women in marginalised bodies (plus-size women, disabled women and black women, especially darker-skinned black women) have been excluded from mainstream media representation or, when they have been included in things like TV and film, they've been made a mockery of.

A study published in the journal *Obesity* (2003), which analysed 238 episodes from popular TV shows, found that overweight characters were more likely to be portrayed as lazy, unattractive and lacking in self-control. Another study, published in the journal *Health Communication*, found that fat characters in films were more likely to be portrayed as socially inferior, less successful and less happy than their thinner counterparts. This study analysed 100 films made from 1991 to 2000 and found that larger-bodied characters were often used as comedic foils or portrayed as pathetic losers.

Up until very recently, the level of diversity we've seen in the media in terms of body shapes and sizes was essentially zero. And although so many people are now talking about diversity, I've only noticed a very small shift in the way women's bodies are actually being presented in the media. This is as sad as it is frustrating, and here's why:

- Firstly, because we can all too easily internalise the media's narrow and unrealistic beauty ideals and start judging ourselves and our own appearance through the same attenuated lens.
- Secondly, because we can all too easily come to believe that being attractive is what matters most in this world. When we watch TV or scroll Instagram, we don't just see beautiful people. We see how other people *treat* them. We see how beauty is praised as if it were a major achievement, we see that more conventionally attractive

Instagrammers have the biggest followings, and we see that leading ladies in the latest films tend to have tiny silhouettes and perfectly symmetrical faces.

THE "HEADLESS FATTY"

A subtle but pervasive way the media reinforces the stereotypes that fat people have to confront daily is the use of images of fat bodies with their heads cropped off. This is so pervasive, in fact, that such images actually have a name: the "headless fatty".

You know the ones I'm talking about. We see them on the evening news whenever there is talk of the nation's growing "obesity epidemic". It's normally a still image – or, if we're really lucky, a video – of a headless individual, wearing a top that's too small for them, walking down the high street. Extra bonus points if they're carrying food; even better if they're lifting it towards their mouths!

This type of imagery has been criticised by activists and public health researchers for almost a decade now. And yet here we are, still seeing them on every prime-time news bulletin and in every newspaper whenever obesity or fatness is mentioned.

These images contribute to the stigmatisation of fat people in a way that would be completely unacceptable in other public health contexts. Can you imagine, for example, the equivalent pictures being used with a HIV/AIDS story today?

People will often try and defend "headless fatty" images under the guise of respecting the person's identity – the idea being "What face would want to be identified as belonging to that body?" Another – kinder, though still misguided – defence is that they are "protecting" the person, in the same way we might obscure a child's face in a newspaper story.

But removing a person's head reduces their humanity. It makes them a mere body-object that can be abstractly discussed, ridiculed and abused. These images stigmatise by reducing a person to being to a single trait. They quite literally, as well as symbolically, decapitate them.

"When we reduce fat people to their bodies, to 'before and after', or to bellies and rolls," says fat activist Aubrey Gordon in her book *What We Don't Talk About When We Talk About Fat*, "we come to think of fat people as bodies without personhood." As such, fat bodies become "symbols of disembodied disgust".

A NOTE ON THE "OBESITY EPIDEMIC"

Another bone of contention I have with traditional media is how it talks about, and reports on, the so-called "obesity epidemic". We're constantly told that we're getting fatter by the day, and that this is a crisis that requires drastic intervention. But is this really the case, or are we being misled by scaremongering headlines and distorted statistics?

First, let's take a look at what we mean by "obesity". The term itself has come to be fraught with judgement and stigma, often being used to imply that larger-bodied individuals are to blame for their own health problems. This ignores the systemic factors that often contribute to weight gain, such as poverty and lack of access to healthcare. It also ignores that weight is not always under an individual's control, diets and exercise are not always effective in achieving weight loss in the long term, and there is no one-size-fits-all definition of what constitutes a "healthy" weight (more on this later, in Chapter 6).

Another common media tactic is to present statistics out of context to exaggerate the scale of the supposed epidemic. For example, we're often told two-thirds of Americans are overweight or obese, implying the vast majority of that population is at risk of serious health problems. However, this statistic is based on the flawed BMI (body mass index) measurement, which has been shown to be an inaccurate and unreliable indicator of health (again, more on this later, in Chapter 6).

Plus, they also often focus on individual cases of extreme obesity, presenting them as representative of the population as a whole. These "shock" stories, such as those about the "half-ton man" or the "world's fattest woman", are designed to elicit a visceral reaction of disgust and fear, rather than provide accurate information about health or weight.

THE MAGIC OF MAKEOVER SHOWS

I don't know about you, but as a teenager I was obsessed with reality TV and transformation shows, such as *10 Years Younger, Supersize vs Superskinny* and *America's Next Top Model*. If I'm honest, I think they gave me hope that one day I, too, could transform from an "ugly duckling" into a "beautiful swan".

Funnily enough, there was actually a US show called *The Swan* that my mum and I would watch together religiously. If you haven't heard of it, the show followed a group of "ordinary" women deemed to be unattractive and suffering from low self-esteem, and gave them all extreme makeovers with specially selected plastic surgeons. Each of them was put through a brutal three-month makeover for the chance to become beauty queens. Each week, two contestants were transformed, but only one would be judged beautiful enough to move on to the pageant at the end. Even writing this gives me the ick.

Season One contestant Lorrie Arias, who was 34 when she went on the series back in 2004, was given a tummy tuck, buttock lift, inner thigh lift, dual facelift, upper lip lift, upper and lower eye lift, endoscopic brow lift, rhinoplasty, breast augmentation and breast lift. In 2010, Arias said she regained all the weight she lost in the aftermath of the series, and became depressed, bipolar and agoraphobic, suffering from body dysmorphic disorder.

Other contestants have also spoken out about how horrendous the show was, and its lack of aftercare. It's fair to say that, like a lot of '90s TV shows, The Swan really didn't age well. But the most toxic of them all, I would argue, was The Biggest Loser. This show ran for 13 seasons in the US, finishing in only 2020, and promised viewers dramatic weight-loss transformations week after week. Each season, filmed over the course of about six months, pushed its contestants to lose as much weight as possible, as quickly as they could. Whoever lost the most weight would win a massive $250,000 prize and the title of "Biggest Loser".

To achieve such dramatic results, the contestants were placed on very low-calorie diets (sometimes under 1,000 calories per day), and were put through strenuous six-hour workouts, often resulting in the contestants fainting or being sick, or both. Trainers Bob Harper and Jillian Michaels repeatedly shouted at contestants as they exercised. Some of Michaels' most infamous statements have included: "I'm proud that I made him vomit"; "I don't care if people die on this floor – you better die looking good"; "It's fun watching other people suffer like that".

One contestant, Tracey Yukich, was airlifted to a hospital after a workout. Another stopped eating altogether and urinated blood. Another suffered multiple stress fractures in her feet, but was still forced to run by producers.

Kai Hibbard, who was runner-up on Season Three after losing an alarming 8.4 stone (118 lb/53 kg) in just 12 weeks, now cites The Biggest Loser as the cause of her eating disorder. This, she says, also led to major hair loss and amenorrhea (her periods stopping), and nearly cost her life. All for our viewing pleasure!

Not only did the majority of contestants regain a significant amount (if not all) of the weight lost during the show, but some were also left with permanent damage to their metabolisms because of the repeated loss and gain of significant amounts of weight (also known as weight cycling), meaning their bodies actually burn up to 800 fewer calories per day than they did before.

And it's not just the contestants who suffered. How many of us still consider exercise a punishment because of this show, or others like it? Or think that unless we're bent over puking and at the point of collapse, we're not working out hard enough?

As far as I'm concerned, fat people face enough stigma in their day-to-day lives without the influence of these detrimental shows. The only good thing to come out of all this is the growing collective horror as we look back and realise how ghastly these shows really were, which says to me that things are at least moving in the right direction – albeit slowly.

WHY ARE WE ALWAYS "THE FAT, FUNNY ONES"?

When you think about your favourite fat characters in TV and film, are they the funny best friend? Is weight or weight loss the central component of their story or character? Do they spend most of their screen time trying to prove they deserve love or friendship despite their size? If your answer to any of these questions is yes, you've discovered the tropes these characters are relegated to whenever Hollywood wants to explore the fat experience.

Honestly, this never occurred to me when I was younger. I just accepted them as gospel. But the truth is that for decades, TV and film have normalised bullying fat people.

Have you noticed that if, by some miracle, fat people are afforded a role, their entire personality is often based on their weight, with them very rarely being given a complex character arc?

In *Friends,* when the storyline cuts back in time to "Fat Monica", she plays right into fat stereotypes, like always having food in her hand or eating sloppily, or she's portrayed as this monstrosity that could only be happy if she loses weight. Not only that, but her entire personality as "Fat Monica" is different from the slim version of her – she's shown as clumsy, stupid, shy and lazy. Even in the alternate timeline the show explored, in which Monica doesn't ever lose weight, she's still an object of humiliation.

Growing up, I really liked *Friends*. And I guess you could say it was just of its time. But I also think it's a demonstration of lazy writing. The same can be said for the movie *The Whale*, released in 2022. If you haven't seen it, the film revolves around a 600-pound (270-kg) gay man called Charlie who hides in his apartment and binge-eats because he's depressed that the love of his life, Alan, died by suicide. When we first meet Charlie, he is sinking into his dirty couch, surrounded by rubbish and masturbating to pornography. I don't want to give away any spoilers, but let's just say life is far from rosy for him.

What frustrated me so much about the film is that it represents a distorted depiction of fatness as a form of squalor. Charlie is a stereotypical caricature who reinforces the belief that fat individuals bring this upon themselves – that we mindlessly devour buckets of fried chicken and push away any chance of love and happiness. In my opinion, there was no joy in the film whatsoever, and I think the only reason some people responded positively to it is because it confirms their biases about what fat people are like.

Another thing that really irritates me in TV and film is how, more often than not, the idea of weight gain or becoming fat is treated as the worst thing in the world.

In the *Sex and the City* movie, when Samantha arrives for Charlotte's baby shower, all the group can talk about is her gut and how much weight she's gained (which, spoiler alert, was only about 5 pounds (2 kg), and was only achieved by the actress, Kim Cattrall, being put in a costume a size too small for her). To make matters worse, Samantha is then seen "eating her feelings" while her supposed best friends take food off her and talk like her weight gain is the end of the world. Even though Carrie says, "This isn't about the weight; you would look gorgeous at any size," her initial reaction definitely says otherwise.

Treating weight gain or the idea of being fat as a social death sentence makes people think that fat people cannot be happy and exist as they are, and it sucks.

A recent example is Netflix's *Isn't It Romantic*, in which Rebel Wilson's character Natalie grows up dreaming that one day her life can be like a romcom. It isn't until after an incident with a mugger, during which she hits her head, that she ascends into a stereotypical romcom reality. Is it really that far-fetched for someone like Liam Hemsworth to fall for Rebel Wilson? It sends the message that the only way to find love is by losing weight or getting a head injury. No, thanks.

Fortunately, there has been some positive representation in recent years. Hulu's *Shrill* (based on the book by Lindy West) follows an up-and-coming journalist at an alternative magazine who is bright, talented and fat. This show unpacks internalised fatphobia and the attendant "smaller body, bigger life" narrative, which I love.

As a huge *This Is Us* fan, I also love the fact they changed the story arc of Kate (played by the fabulous Chrissy Metz) after the first couple of seasons, to not be just about her weight, her self-loathing and her inability to even *want* to love, let alone find it. Instead, they focus on her pursuit of becoming a professional singer, raising her young family and her marital problems.

The sceptic in me thinks that the TV and film industry must be out to normalise body hatred for anyone who lacks supermodel proportions. But wouldn't it be great to see a large-bodied female lead whose storyline has nothing to do with her size, weight or appearance? Instead, it's just her, living her best life? Is that really too much to ask?

WHY WE NEED A PLUS-SIZE DISNEY PRINCESS

In recent years, the push for greater representation and inclusivity in popular culture has been gaining momentum. From race to gender to body size, people are advocating for more diverse and realistic portrayals of individuals across all media platforms. The world of Disney princesses, however, remains largely homogeneous, with a glaring omission: a plus-size princess.

The lack of a plus-size princess is not only a failure to accurately represent the diverse range of body sizes in our society, but also a missed opportunity to promote body positivity and self-love to young audiences.

A plus-size princess would lessen the stigma often associated with being the fat kid. It would show young girls and boys they can be valued, loved and successful regardless of their size.

The fatter (and thus "uglier") characters tend to be the villains or the comic relief in Disney films; for example, Ursula in *The Little Mermaid*, Governor Ratcliffe in *Pocahontas,* and Hades in *Hercules.* And while the thin and beautiful characters get the happy ending, the fat and unconventional, for the most part, don't.

A 2014 analysis of popular children's movies conducted by researchers at the University of North Carolina at Chapel Hill found that larger-bodied characters were more likely to be depicted as villains or comedic sidekicks, reinforcing negative stereotypes and stigma against plus-size people. The study analysed 81 movies released between 2006 and 2010, and also found that larger characters were often portrayed as clumsy, lazy or lacking in self-control.

It did seem like things were changing when, in 2022, Disney finally introduced us to our first plus-size protagonist in *Reflect* – a six-minute animated short which welcomes young ballet dancer Bianca to the small screen. She's passionate about the craft, but appears disappointed when she sees her reflection in the mirror, sucking in her belly and lifting her chin up to fit in. Straight away, Bianca is transported to a barely lit room, where mirrors reign supreme and the young dancer comes face to face with her reflection at all angles. This, of course, is meant to symbolise the body dysmorphia she's experiencing. Fortunately, Bianca's love for dance trumps her feelings of inferiority, as each of her swift dance moves shatters the reflection she had been criticising earlier.

Overall, the reception for *Reflect* was positive. But the question remains: why must Disney's first plus-size main character be featured in a story that solely focuses on body image? The fat experience is so much more than just the fatphobia we experience. This doesn't feel like true representation.

It's definitely a step forward, yes. I think it's important we celebrate this as progress while also recognising it took far too long to get here, and it's still not enough. Bianca is not a Disney princess, and the film was only six minutes long. We can only hope that, with time, we'll have an overwhelming amount of media to choose from that not only highlights characters of all genders, sizes, abilities and races, but does so in a well-rounded, relatable way.

Just think how incredible it would be if, instead of saying "I want to look like her", young girls could watch their favourite Disney film and say: "She looks like me."

This is exactly what happened when we found out a black actress was taking on the role of Ariel in the 2023 live-action remake of *The Little Mermaid*, with young girls all over the world seeing themselves represented for perhaps the first time. Their emotional response was compelling, and just goes to show the power of representation.

UNDERSTANDING SOCIAL MEDIA AND BODY IMAGE

A decade ago, everyone was talking about how Photoshop was affecting body image. This led to people, even models, calling out magazines for being a bit too slap-happy with the smoother tool. "Even I want to wake up looking like Cindy Crawford," supermodel Cindy Crawford is famously quoted as saying.

Now, with the ever-growing popularity of social media, it's not Photoshop we have to worry about, but filters. These filters allow us to alter our appearance in real time, making us look more polished, slimmer, more symmetrical.

It seems that the days of the Snapchat "dog filter" have been replaced by a dystopian reality – and this genuinely scares me. More than 50% of girls believe they don't look "good enough" without photo editing, according to the Dove Self-Esteem Project. And 67% of girls try to change or hide at least one body part/feature before posting a photo of themselves on social media.

In 2023, a filter called "Bold Glamour" launched on TikTok. It's a sophisticated AI technology that manipulates a user's features to provide a digital "fix". Once applied, users are fitted with hollowed cheekbones, narrower noses, pore-free skin, razor-sharp eyebrows and enough contour for the population of Europe. It can look so realistic, and a lot of users are saying it should be banned.

I tried it and I didn't like it, but what I found upsetting was being faced with my natural bare skin afterwards. In truth, it made me feel ugly and dissatisfied. It's no surprise, then, that the use of filters like this on social media are often linked to the rise of low self-esteem, negative body image, body dysmorphia, eating disorders, anxiety and depression.

The use of filters can also create an unhealthy obsession with perfection, causing us to focus on the tiniest of "flaws" and leading to a constant need to improve our appearance – which can be especially harmful to young people who are still developing their sense of self.

It's also worth noting that filters are often based on Eurocentric beauty standards, which, as discussed in Chapter 3, can reinforce the idea that there is only one acceptable way to look and can lead to feelings of shame or inadequacy among those who don't fit into that exclusionary standard.

CRUEL COMPARISONS: THE DARK SIDE OF SOCIAL MEDIA

Sometimes it can feel like the internet is divided into two halves. For every person banging on about the need for calorie deficits, there's another telling us to love our bodies just as they are. On the whole, I think social media can be a force for good, providing that you curate your own news feed (more on this in Chapter 8). But there is a dark side to it that can impact our mental health and our body image.

It's important to note that research into social media and body image is still in its early stages, so it hasn't yet been proven whether a platform such as Facebook, for example, causes someone to have negative feelings about their appearance, or whether people who are concerned about their appearance are more likely to use Facebook.

That said, using social media does appear to be correlated with body-image concerns. A systematic review of 20 papers published in 2016 found that photo-based activities, like scrolling through Instagram or posting pictures of yourself, were a particular problem when it came to negative thoughts about your body.

Another of my pet peeves when it comes to social media are the prolific "What I eat in a day" videos, which involve an influencer sharing a breakdown of their meals, including their protein, carb and fat intake, and how they achieve it daily. Many of these start with said influencer posting a photo or video of their body to show their "progress" earned as a result of their diet. Often, they're wearing tight clothing to show off their thin body, and/or pulling in their stomach muscles and posing in a way that makes them look smaller.

What worries me about this is that people, particularly young people, think if they can copy the behaviours of someone who they find attractive, they will somehow look the same. Even if the words "weight" or "calories" aren't mentioned, the visual image of a smaller-bodied person talking about food and exercise is enough to lead some people to compare themselves to it.

Many of these posts also tend to moralise food using health buzzwords such as "clean eating" or other food terms related to pseudoscience or misleading diet trends. The worst part is that such videos have been proven to influence teenagers and trigger people with a history of disordered eating or eating disorders. So, while they may seem harmless, or annoying at best, they're anything but.

My other big gripe with social media has to be "before and after" photos. We've all seen them. On the left is a pale, hunched-over woman, un-posed in an ill-fitting bikini, standing in a room with harsh lighting, looking really sad. On the right is a polished, perfectly manicured "picture of health", one leg in front of the other, hips back, designer bikini, huge grin and newly whitened teeth. I hate them almost as much as I hate the "If I can do it, so can you" caption that often lurks underneath them.

I get that people want to celebrate their weight-loss or fitness journey. I do. But (and it's a big but) when you are twice, or even three times, the size of the person in the "before" photo, it makes you feel pretty shitty about your own body, like you're not even good enough to be a before photo.

The other issue with before and after photos is that they often promise a quick fix to all of our body-image woes – a way to transform ourselves into the "perfect" version of ourselves.

Before and after photos exist in every corner of social media, but they're most pervasive in the weight-loss space. Often, these posts elicit comments that seem positive, like, "so inspiring!" or "you look great!" But there's a flip side to these comments: the implication is that the person didn't look great in their larger body, and so being thinner is always better.

Such messages, whether subtle or overt, contribute to weight stigma and anti-fat bias, and perpetuate the notion that we're simply not good enough as we are, and that changing our body, losing weight or being thinner is the only way to "fix" ourselves and feel happy – when the truth is that our bodies are constantly changing, and that's OK. We should be celebrating our bodies at *every* stage of our lives, not just when we reach some arbitrary ideal.

BUT THINGS ARE CHANGING, RIGHT?

We've come a long way since the early 2000s, with Fat Bastard in the Austin Powers films and whatever the hell was going on in *Shallow Hal*. Social media is now *mostly* good (depending on the platform), and we now have plus-size models and more representation in the music charts. BUT they're still very much the exception and not the rule. There's much work yet to be done.

In New York Fashion Week 2023, over 3,000 models graced the catwalk. Only 30 of them were considered plus size. That's 1%. And most of that 1% weren't even *technically* "plus size" (i.e. bigger than a UK size 18, or US size 14). They were just a larger size than your average model, plus they happened to be impossibly tall, with hourglass figures, which meant that even *their* frames aren't exactly attainable to your average Joe!

Friends in the fashion industry also tell me that the vast majority of "plus-size" models use implants, liposuction and fat-transfer procedures to ensure they have "curves in all the right places" in order to be deemed acceptable by brands. And that some of the smaller "plus-size" models are even made to wear fat suits, or padding, at times. Why? Because brands still want them to have a chiselled jaw, apparently! Sigh.

There is also a huge issue with tokenism in the fashion industry. This is essentially the act of including one or two members of a marginalised group, such as plus-size models or models of colour, in a project, campaign or event solely for the purpose of appearing diverse and inclusive. While this may seem like progress, it's superficial and does nothing to address the underlying issues of systemic inequality and discrimination. It's like putting a Band-Aid on a bullet wound. Sure, it may look better, but it's not actually solving the problem.

You might want to think of it like inviting a "diverse" friend to dinner parties only to make your group look better or more interesting. But the person is then not given much chance to speak, their opinions are often overlooked and they're constantly reminded, whether overtly or subtly, of their "otherness".

True progress would require a commitment to diversity and inclusion at all levels of the industry, from the design room to the runway. I think a lot of brands struggle when it comes to designing clothes for plus-size women because they don't have people like this in their buying or design teams, which means that they have no true fat perspective. (Side note: just think how much better the clothes would be and how much companies would save in clothing returns if they changed this!)

Tokenism not only fails to address the root causes of the fashion industry's lack of diversity, but it also perpetuates harmful stereotypes and reinforces the idea that only certain types of people belong in that "beautiful" world.

The industry has simply got to do better. It needs to commit to substantial change by actively seeking out and hiring diverse talent at all levels, creating opportunities for under-represented groups, and working to dismantle the systemic barriers that prevent marginalised communities from entering and succeeding in that world.

Having one plus-size model among a group of straight-size models (as they're known) is better than nothing at all, but we want to see plus-size models with lots of different body shapes, models with disabilities, mature models …

At a basic level, I think every woman deserves to be able to see a dress, or any other garment that we like, modelled by someone who has a similar body type to us – to remind us that we, too, can wear the beautiful things being displayed and we, too, *are* beautiful and deserve to be seen as such.

WHAT ABOUT MALE BODY IDEALS?

While weight stigma impacts us all, as we were exploring in Chapter 2, I think we can safely say that women are disproportionately affected by it. I think this is as a result of an intersection with misogyny, which is, unfortunately, a deeply rooted part of a traditional, conservative patriarchal society that dictates women have to be attractive to find a partner, get married and start a family, etc.

However, just like Disney princesses don't have cellulite (or chin hair, or a FUPA – "fat upper pussy area", in case you didn't know), male superheroes don't have love handles (or receding hairlines, or acne scars). The alpha males we see in the media are pretty much always portrayed as tall and strong, with a chiselled jaw, full head of hair and a symmetrical face. Ideally, they also have a large penis and no "man boobs"!

Just like women, then, men are often faced with depictions in the media about how they "should" look. There are sleek fitness hunks everywhere: on billboards and in magazines, in TV ads and in shopping windows. And I imagine that this image of what masculinity "should" look like has been burned into the collective consciousness of a lot of men – resulting, no doubt, in a lot of male body-image issues that run much deeper than just weight.

The underlying notion that guys, too, need to "improve" their bodies has meant an upswing in the number of social media posts about male fitness, male celebrity "transformations" and even male cosmetic surgeries.

One of the main challenges when it comes to the self-image issues that men are now facing is simply that not enough people seem to be talking about or doing much work to make it better.

My wish is that we start to more widely acknowledge the fact that men face their own distinct challenges when it comes to body image. By breaking down the stigma surrounding discussions of male body image and promoting more diverse representations of male bodies, as well as female bodies, in the media, we can be hugely instrumental in making men feel more comfortable in their own skin.

SO WHERE DO WE GO FROM HERE?

As already touched on, the film and TV industries have traditionally, and often, portrayed fat people in one of two ways: either as lazy, unattractive losers who are the butt of every joke, or as loveable sidekicks who exist solely to support and uplift the thin, conventionally attractive main character. While there's certainly nothing wrong with being a supportive mate, it's high time we saw some fat people in leading roles.

It's time to move beyond the tired trope of the fat best friend. Fat people are, after all, so much more than that. Believe it or not, we, too, have dreams, ambitions and desires, just like everyone else. We, too, are capable of being heroes, villains and everything in between.

It's time for the media to stop perpetuating the idea that fatness is inherently unattractive or unhealthy. Contrary to popular belief, you *can* be both fat and healthy, and you *can* be both fat and beautiful.

So it's time to demand more from the media. It's time to call out fatphobic jokes and storylines when we see them, and to push for more nuanced and authentic representations of fat people in all forms of media. It's also time to support fat creators and artists, who are often pushing the boundaries of what it means to be fat in our society.

Fat representation in the media is about more than just being able to see people who look like us on screen. It's also about dismantling harmful stereotypes and changing the way our society thinks about, and treats, fat people. And hey, if we can get more fat leading ladies and action heroes out of it, that's the much-deserved cherry on top.

SELF-EMPOWERMENT TASK

We can't control what traditional media sources, such as newspapers and television, present to us. But we can, to some extent, control which of these we choose to buy and watch, and what we choose to view online.

So, take some time to become more aware of what media sources you habitually expose yourself to, and start curating your social media feed more mindfully by following more people who look like you (as well as people who don't) and by unfollowing anyone who makes you feel bad or who you follow just because you like the way they look.

5

The unbearable weight of diet culture

What it is and why it's so damaging

Years ago, before every weekly weigh-in at Slimming World, my mum and I would pretty much starve ourselves in the hope of losing a couple of pounds that week. Carbs were off limits, and even water was kept to a minimum. Oh, and let's not forget about the obligatory pre-weigh-in wee (a poo if you were *really* lucky).

Every week, like clockwork, we'd step on the scale, hold our breath and wait to see the little numbers pop up. And every week after our weigh-in, just like clockwork, we'd reward ourselves with a treat (usually something beige or deep-fried).

I remember one week we came home and I scoffed down a sausage sandwich with brown sauce. I can still feel the bread all sticky and warm on the roof of my mouth. About halfway through, I had a brainwave: I realised the sandwich wasn't actually that "bad" according to Slimming World's rules, but that the reason it tasted so good was because it *felt* as if it was off limits.

Have you ever noticed, when you diet, how hard it is to *not* think constantly about food – and that you often count down the hours until you can eat again? Sometimes the cravings get too much and you might "fall off the wagon"? If this sounds familiar, please know that it's not "bad" or a sign of weakness, as Western "diet culture" would have us believe. It is, in fact, a natural physiological response to restriction.

So, what exactly is diet culture, and why does it make us believe things like this? While the diet *industry* sells products and services for weight loss, diet *culture* is what makes us want to buy it in the first place. It is what makes us feel like we *need* to be a certain size or look a certain way in order to have value.

Diet culture is a societal and cultural phenomenon that promotes the idea that being thin or having a certain body type is the ideal standard of beauty and health. It creates the voice in your head that tells you you're not thin enough, not toned enough, not loveable enough, not worthy enough. It's the reason you may have tried every fad diet under the sun and still can't seem to lose weight.

At its core, diet culture is a set of beliefs and practices that equate thinness with health, beauty and moral superiority. As such, it encourages people to restrict their food intake, and to engage in extreme exercise and other harmful behaviours to achieve an idealised body shape.

Diet culture seems to me like a bad houseguest – one who shows up uninvited, makes a mess of everything and then refuses to leave even when it's obvious it's not wanted. This gets exhausting, and is often particularly tough to deal with around Christmas and the New Year.

As soon as the Christmas Day feast gives way to the Boxing Day leftovers, we're bombarded with messages urging us to rid our bodies of all the "bad" foods we've been encouraged to consume during the holidays! Gym membership deals pop up on every high street, Slimming World posters appear through our letterbox, and talk of "burning off" and "making up for" is on everyone's lips in the office. And don't get me started on some influencers selling their fitness and "nutrition" plans before we've even had time to digest our sprouts!

Even as we make the promises to ourselves about how we're going to lose weight, get fit, tone up and "shred" our way into the New Year, we're already feeling guilty about how much we've eaten and drunk over the holiday season. Although that guilt can be a powerful motivator, it usually only serves as such for a short time, ultimately leaving us feeling shame when our new lifestyle plans don't work out. Then it starts all over again, either throughout the year, or the following year – an endless cycle of restriction followed by bingeing. That cycle is so ubiquitous, we often don't even realise how much we're being bombarded with it. It's time to call BS on the all-encompassing effect of diet culture.

WHY IS DIET CULTURE SO DAMAGING?

Diet culture perpetuates the belief that weight loss is a necessary goal – the key to happiness, success and self-worth. It can be seen in the numerous fad diets, weight-loss programmes and fitness regimens that flood the market, all promising quick results and a "perfect" body. And, unfortunately, it often ignores the importance of overall health and wellbeing, instead preying on, and profiting from, our insecurities.

Diet culture tells us that we're not good enough unless we look or eat a certain way, which can lead to restrictive or binge-eating behaviours, eating disorders, self-esteem issues, body dysmorphia, and a host of other mental and physical health issues. But the diet industry doesn't seem to care about that. It cares about selling its products and making a profit. It's a £56 ($70) billion industry based on us hating ourselves. Yes, a whole industry is built on the basis of people's "failures" – which, when you think about it, is pretty fucked up.

A "DAY IN THE LIFE" WITH TOXIC MESSAGING

If you're not yet convinced that diet culture exists, let's run through the toxic messaging I could consume in just a single day:

7am I wake up, let the dog out for a wee and scroll Instagram. I see a suggested post from a reality TV star promoting their new fad diet and exercise programme that has nothing to do with health and everything to do with profiting off of people's insecurities. I read the comments underneath from women who say they feel inspired and have immediately signed up because they want to look like her, with hashtags like #thinspo thrown in for good measure.

8am I make a cuppa and switch on the TV, and watch as four thin people talk about the pros of a "revolutionary" new weight-loss drug that could be a miracle cure for fat people and put an end to the obesity epidemic, which is crippling the healthcare industry.

10am I'm in the office and a colleague tells me she's been "bad" all weekend, so needs to be "good" today by only drinking coffee.

12pm I go to an aqua aerobics class on my lunch break. The instructor tells us we need to work harder to "burn those calories" and "fight the flab".

1pm I'm in the changing rooms after the class and I overhear a group of women talking about what they want for lunch, and how carbs are the enemy.

1.20pm On my way out, I spot a sign about "shredding for the wedding" and how the gym's new weight-loss programme can help brides-to-be drop a dress size before the big day.

3pm Back at the office, an email circulates about a new weight-loss challenge that comprises weekly weigh-ins for accountability. The person who loses the most weight that week wins a prize.

6pm I go shopping and see a campaign in a store window saying "Jeans for EVERYbody". I rush in with excitement but am immediately met with disappointment, as I discover from a sales assistant "EVERYbody" means up to a UK size 22 (US size 18). She suggests I look at their Curve range, which is now exclusively online.

7pm I sit down with my husband to watch a new comedy on Netflix, which is full to the brim with fat jokes.

9pm I wind down for the evening, scroll TikTok and see prank after prank trying to humiliate fat people, women talking about their weight-loss journeys resulting from a new injection that all the celebrities are using, and vile comments underneath my videos, as well as those of other fat content creators, telling us how we're going to get diabetes and die.

Obviously, the above is an exaggerated version of a normal "day in the life", but you get the gist. The impact of diet culture is everywhere, and it's gruelling.

A BRIEF HISTORY OF DIETS

The history of diet culture is, to me, equal parts fascinating and concerning.

In ancient times, diets varied greatly depending on where you lived and what resources were available. In ancient Greece and Rome, for example, a balanced diet was considered essential for good health, so included plenty of fruits, vegetables, grains and meats. Meanwhile, in medieval Europe, the diet was much more limited, with the average person surviving on a diet of bread, porridge and perhaps a little meat if they were lucky.

The 1600s saw the rise of "deprivation diets", where people would fast or eat only a limited selection of foods in an attempt to improve their health. The idea was to rid the body of toxins and impurities.

With the Industrial Revolution came the rise of middle-class leisure time, during which diets shifted more towards vanity. The "take small bites" diet was all the rage in the 1800s, with people advised to eat less and exercise more. This idea was taken to new extremes in the 1920s with the flapper craze, where thin meant fashionable.

The 20th century saw a proliferation of fad diets, from the Grapefruit Diet to the Cabbage Soup Diet. But it wasn't until the 1970s that diets really hit the mainstream. In 1972, Dr Robert Atkins published *Dr. Atkins' Diet Revolution*, introducing the world to the low-carb, high-fat Atkins Diet. This was a radical departure from the low-fat diets of the previous decade and sparked a trend that has continued until today, when fat is now seen by many as "good", and carbs are the enemy.

The 1980s saw the rise of weight-loss supplements and meal-replacement drinks, such as SlimFast. The focus was on quick and easy weight loss, but the long-term health benefits were often questionable.

The 1990s saw the emergence of the Zone Diet, which put an emphasis on portion control and the right balance of carbohydrates, proteins and fats, and also the South Beach Diet, which offered a similar approach to weight loss.

And then came the 2000s – a time of low-rise jeans, flip phones and some seriously dubious diet trends.

First came the juice cleanse, which involved consuming nothing but cold-pressed juices for days on end, in the belief it would "detox" your body and leave you feeling like a new person. In reality, it left you feeling hungry, irritable and with a serious case of juice-induced flatulence.

Next came the gluten-free diet. This started as a way to manage coeliac disease, but quickly turned into a fad diet for anyone who wanted to appear healthier. Suddenly, everything from pizza to beer was being marketed as gluten-free, despite the fact most people had no idea what gluten even was.

But perhaps the most infamous diet of the 2000s was the Atkins Diet, which saw a resurgence since its introduction in the '70s. Suddenly, everyone was eating bacon-wrapped cheeseburgers and claiming it was for their health.

In more recent years, we've seen the rise of the paleo diet and the keto diet. The paleo diet is all about eating like our caveman ancestors, which means cutting out processed foods and loading up on meat and vegetables. The keto diet involves consuming high amounts of fat and cutting out carbs and sugar to achieve ketosis – a metabolic state in which the body burns fat, instead of carbohydrates, for fuel.

Intermittent fasting became the new buzzword in the health and wellness industry in the mid-2010s, which is funny to me, as people have been fasting for centuries, whether it's for religious or cultural reasons. So, why the sudden hype? Probably because influencers and celebrities alike were seen touting the benefits of it, which suddenly made it the hottest thing on the planet. But we seem to forget that just because someone has a million followers on Instagram, it doesn't mean they're a health expert! Plus, the benefits of intermittent fasting have been blown way out of proportion. Yes, there are some potential health benefits, but there are doubts as to whether they're as ground-breaking as some would have you believe. And let's not forget that fasting can have some serious side effects, such as fatigue, headaches and irritability.

The main problem with all these fad diets and trends is that they tend to promise quick fixes and overnight results, yet sustainable weight loss and a healthy lifestyle don't happen overnight.

You'd have thought we'd have learnt our lesson by this stage, but no. Throughout the late 2010s we were witness to thousands of influencers and reality TV stars promoting laxative teas and "Skinny Jab" weight-loss injections on social media.

In 2016, a new app called Noom emerged as an alternative to traditional diets. It garnered a significant following of over 50 million users by offering sustainable results and a healthier approach to food. However, despite the app's "no dieting needed" marketing and claim of being created by psychologists and backed by scientific research, when I looked more closely at it, it felt, in my opinion, like just another diet. It seems to me that Noom is, essentially, a slightly tweaked version of a calorie tracker – but accompanied by online lessons on behaviour change, and a personal coach who provides messages of support. And while the personalised coaching feature of Noom might seem beneficial, as far as I'm concerned, the app's heavy reliance on restricting certain foods could still promote an unhealthy relationship with food and eating.

WHY DIETS DON'T WORK

Dieting is a multi-billion-dollar industry, with countless books, products and programmes promising quick and easy weight loss. But the truth is, we've been lied to our whole lives. Diets just don't work. So, why is this? Let's take a look:

The problem with calorie restriction

Being in a calorie deficit (i.e. eating fewer calories than you're burning) is often seen as the holy grail of weight loss; the idea is that this is how weight loss technically happens. But, unfortunately, it's not all it's cracked up to be.

Firstly, let's address the elephant in the room: cutting back on your favourite foods and constantly monitoring your intake is a recipe for misery. Sure, you may lose weight in the short term, but at what cost? Your social life? Your sanity?

It's not just the psychological toll of calorie restriction that's the problem. There are physical consequences, too. When you drastically reduce your calorie intake, your body goes into survival mode, slowing down your metabolism to conserve energy. This can lead to a weight-loss plateau, making it even harder to lose weight.

NHS doctor, nutritionist and author Dr Joshua Wolrich says that repeated attempts at weight loss, or cycles of losing and gaining weight, have been shown to lead to fat being stored in areas that are harder to lose. This is because losing weight can disrupt, or even stop, important biological processes like periods, which can negatively impact the body's ability to reproduce. As such, weight loss is actually seen as harmful by the body, which means it may start to compensate by putting on more weight.

"It's important to understand that the human body is designed to protect itself." says Dr Wolrich. "Our bodies are not designed to constantly lose weight and keep it off. Instead, our bodies are designed to thrive, and this is something we should consider when discussing body size and finding solutions to support people's health."

In addition to accidentally causing your body to retain weight, calorie restriction can sometimes lead to nutrient deficiencies, as you may be depriving your body of the vitamins and minerals it needs to function properly. And let's not forget about the impact on your muscles. When you're not consuming enough protein, your body can begin to break down muscle tissue, leaving you weaker than before.

There's more. Calorie restriction has also been linked to a host of negative mental health outcomes, including increased anxiety and depression. Unsurprisingly, when you're constantly fixated on your intake, and restricted from enjoying the foods you love, it can take a toll on your emotional wellbeing.

Have I mentioned yet that every time I've been on a diet and counting calories, I've been utterly miserable? The deprivation, constant calorie counting and feeling of missing out on social events has always been a very real struggle for me. I remember doing one particularly restrictive diet while at university and my best friend pleading with me after two weeks to just "please eat something" because I was snappy, irritable, had no energy and was generally really unpleasant to be around.

Food makes us happy and is so much more than just calories. So why should we feel restricted or ashamed about eating it and enjoying it in moderation?

The problem with "diet mentality"

Diet mentality – by which I mean the constant need to count calories, restrict food groups and obsess over every morsel that passes our lips – is the bane of many a dieter's existence, and for good reason. Although it can manifest in different ways for different people, essentially it can be recognised as an internal dialogue, or "food police", that dictates food choices.

Below are some of the ways in which diet mentality can show up:

- Compensating for consuming a "bad" food by exercising more, intentionally eating less at subsequent meals, or skipping meals
- Creating specific conditions around eating, such as only allowing oneself to eat a particular food once a month or on designated "cheat days", or restricting carbohydrates after consuming something like a bagel for breakfast
- Using deceptive techniques to fool hunger, such as curbing appetite with coffee, low-calorie drinks or gum, using appetite suppressants or weight-loss pills or consuming low-calorie snacks instead of a proper meal

Firstly, let's talk about the obvious: the fact that diet mentality sucks the joy out of food. When you're constantly worrying about whether a food is "good" or "bad", or how many calories are in a meal, it can be hard to simply enjoy the act of eating.

But it's not just the enjoyment of food that's at stake. As I touched on already, diet mentality can also lead to disordered-eating behaviours such as bingeing, purging and extreme calorie restriction. This is because, when you're in a state of constant deprivation, your body may rebel, leading you to harmful behaviours that are meant to "make up" for what you've eaten, or not eaten.

According to research published in *The International Journal of Obesity* in 2004, making certain foods "forbidden" results in increased food-related thoughts: the greater the attempt to suppress food-related thoughts, the louder they become.

And let's not forget, of course, about the impact on our mental health. As we know by now, when we're constantly worried about our weight or what we're eating, it can take a toll on our self-esteem and overall sense of wellbeing, and can also cause negative ways of thinking that aren't so helpful. Some of these include:

- **Binary thinking:** This is when you see things as either all good or all bad, with nothing in the middle. This can make you feel like a failure if you're not "perfect" all the time.
- **Absolute thinking:** This is when you think there's only one right way to do something, and everything else is wrong. It can stop you from trying new things or exploring different options.
- **Catastrophic and pessimistic thinking:** This is when you always think the worst thing will happen in any situation, which can be stressful and lead to feeling really worried or down.

None of this is great, is it? I hope you can see by now why I'm not exactly a fan of the diet mentality that's become so prevalent in Western society. Why let food stress us out when it can be a source of joy and nourishment instead?

The one-size-fits-all approach

Another problem with diets is that they're rarely personalised to our individual needs. Most are based on the idea that there's a one-size-fits-all solution to weight loss and health, and that if you just follow a specific set of rules, you'll see results. But the truth is, our bodies are all different: we all have varying metabolisms, genetic predispositions and lifestyles that impact our health and weight. This means that what works for one person may not work for another. We could all eat and exercise the same, and we'd all still look distinct from each other and weigh different amounts.

As I've mentioned before, diets also often fail to address the *underlying* causes of weight gain or health issues, whether they're due to stress, sleep, hormones or medical conditions. Plus, they fail to address the deep-seated reasons *why* people overeat in the first place, and therefore don't offer any emotional support for this, which can lead to a real sense of frustration and shame if and when a diet "fails".

A group of Israeli scientists at the Weizmann Institute of Science conducted a study in 2015 that challenged the notion of a "one-size-fits-all" diet. The study found that people's responses to food varied widely and were affected by factors such as genetics, microbiome composition and lifestyle, which really emphasised the need for *customised* nutrition plans over one-size-fits-all diets.

THE DIET/BINGE CYCLE: A VICIOUS LOOP

The diet/binge cycle – which involves a period of restrictive eating followed by an episode of binge-eating – is a common behaviour pattern in the pursuit of weight loss. Sadly, this cycle can lead to serious physical and mental health problems, such as weight fluctuations, malnutrition, digestive issues, disordered eating habits, anxiety, depression and body dissatisfaction.

This cycle can be broken down into component stages, which you may find useful to know:

1. Shame

Before starting any diet, detox or lifestyle change, it's common to feel a sense of shame. Perhaps you feel ashamed of your body size or because you've eaten "too much" in the past. Maybe you feel guilty about eating "bad" foods or feel you need to control your food intake. These feelings can come from external forces, such as comments from friends or family, or from more personal factors, like your clothes feeling too tight or not feeling comfortable in your own skin.

2. Restriction

To take control of the situation, you begin a diet, start cutting back on certain foods or reducing portions. You may not think of it as a diet. Maybe you're just trying to "clean up" your eating patterns or "cut back" on sugary snacks, for example. But both of those things are a *form* of dieting and/or restriction, as they involve telling yourself not to eat certain things, or to eat less. The restriction is likely to feel challenging at times, but for a few days or weeks, you may feel empowered and in control.

3. Intense cravings

You start to realise that food is consuming your thoughts, like an obsession. You might feel intense cravings for certain "off-limit" foods, or you might feel extreme hunger for any food, even when you've just eaten. You might even start dreaming about food.

4. Bingeing

Eventually, your intense cravings become too much to handle, and you give in to a binge. You may start by eating an "off-limit" food and find that you can't stop. You may feel guilty or out of control, and it's easy to tell yourself that you'll start the diet again tomorrow. For some, the bingeing isn't too intense, but they still feel out of control around food and eat until they're slightly uncomfortable.

It's important to note that bingeing isn't just about the amount of food you eat. There's a psychological component that involves feeling distressed, out of control, guilty or secretive.

5. Back to the start

Then, as you feel shame about your bingeing or lack of control, the cycle begins again and you go back to stage one: shame.

This diet/binge cycle can be a vicious loop that takes a heavy toll on both physical and mental health. If this is something you're struggling with, please know that it's not your fault, and you're not alone.

We'll talk more about how to improve your relationship with food in Chapter 11, but if you find yourself battling this pattern of behaviour consistently, please consider seeking help from a professional such as your GP, a nutritionist or a psychologist.

SO WHAT'S THE ALTERNATIVE
TO DIET CULTURE?

Instead of allowing ourselves to get wrapped up, and bogged down, in the societal construct of diet culture, which tends to focus on weight loss as the ultimate goal, how about we shift our attention to a more holistic sense of health and wellbeing?

A holistic approach to health is all about seeing how various aspects of your life are connected, rather than just focusing on weight, size or physical fitness. It means looking at your physical, mental, emotional *and* social wellbeing in order to identify areas that may need some TLC.

We'll be looking more at the need to define health beyond the scales in the next chapter, and we'll then be covering a whole host of simple but powerful ways in which you can "take back the power" when it comes to your relationship with your own body, including your relationship with eating, in Part 2.

SELF-EMPOWERMENT TASK

Take a little time out for yourself and see if you can identify ways in which "diet mentality" shows up in your own life – whether in the form of a lack of joy and ease when you think about eating, a strong inner "food police" voice about what foods you view as "good" and "bad", or any of the other aspects of diet mentality mentioned above.

You might also want to have a think about any particular "diet culture" *triggers* in your life, whether in the past or now. For example, maybe seeing pictures of skinny models in magazines makes you compare yourself to them and feel like shit, maybe reading about other people's weight-loss "successes" makes you feel like a failure or maybe spending time with particular people drains you of energy because you feel that they judge you as a result of your weight.

Feel free to write down anything that feels particularly powerful and/or that you feel you could do with trying to avoid on a daily basis in order to start escaping from the crippling weight of Western society's diet culture.

6

"But what about health?"
Redefining health beyond the scales

"I'm just concerned about your health."

"I'm all for body positivity, but I don't believe in glorifying obesity."

"I think fat people deserve respect, but it's just not heathy to be bigger."

The "but what about *health*?" question is often a key argument used against body acceptance – and something you might even have been thinking about as you've been reading this book.

There's often an assumption that if we accept our bodies as they are, we'll "give up" on our health and sit on the couch eating nothing but pizza and ice cream all day. There's also a misconception that health is a look (measurable by size) – and that we have total control over our weight. But the truth is much more complex.

In this chapter, with the help of research insights from NHS doctor, nutritionist and author Dr Joshua Wolrich, we're going to look at what health means, how we define it, how we measure it and how it's linked to body image.

My hope is that it helps you to rethink what you've been told about health, and separate your health from the way you look.

HARMFUL ASSUMPTIONS

We live in a society with such a deep-rooted fear of fat that many of us are unwilling to even consider the idea that our weight might not actually define our health. People will often say that they work to stay slim because being slim means being healthy, but I think, a lot of the time, that's just a cover for how scared they really are of the idea of just being fat in a society that doesn't treat that as being aesthetically OK.

Consider this: if you were given the choice between being fat and healthy, or slim and *unhealthy*, which option would you choose? If you hesitated before answering, it highlights my point that things really aren't clear-cut when it comes to the reasons why so many people view fat as "bad".

Therefore, when someone brings up health as a concern in relation to weight, I know that it doesn't *necessarily* mean that they genuinely care about my actual health. To me, it seems that phrases like "but what about health?" are often used as a sort of fallback by some people when their other comments about weight don't seem to be working for them. It's like when people accuse me of "promoting obesity" – as if I spend all day handing out flyers to people on the street, trying to recruit them with McDonald's vouchers or something. In my opinion, even *health*-related comments about weight often reveal deeper, stigmatising beliefs about a person's appearance, abilities, attractiveness and/or worth.

Dr Wolrich agrees: "The assumption that weight defines our health is something we need to be questioning whenever it comes up. It's so engrained that we judge the effectiveness of any health-seeking behaviour based on whether or not it's resulted in weight loss. Take exercise as a perfect example. Regular movement is amazing for your health, but many people will only start doing it because they've been told it will make them lose weight. When this doesn't happen, disillusion sets in and activity levels fall again."

While body size *can*, of course, impact health, it is not the only factor. Other things – like sleep, nutrition, physical activity, exposure to sunlight and how many times we go to the toilet each day – all play a role in our overall health. And this is something that is not spoken about enough.

SO, CAN YOU BE IN A BIGGER BODY AND STILL BE HEALTHY?

"Let's clear up any potential confusion at the start," says Dr Wolrich. "The extremes of body weight, at either end of the spectrum, can have a negative impact on your health. That goes for pretty much everything in life, from drinking water to how much you sleep. Having said that, it can still be very difficult to tease out whether it's actually body fat that's causing a problem or something else. Our health is incredibly multifaceted."

It's really important to acknowledge how complex this all is. We can't just dismiss bigger people as having a lack of self-control or mental health issues. As we've been discussing, the reality is much more nuanced, with a wide variety of factors contributing to an individual's body size – including past experiences of stress, discrimination and stigma, as well as genetics and socio-economic factors, such as food poverty and lack of education about nutrition.

A lot of disordered eating and overeating also stems from trauma. For example, people who suffer sexual abuse at a young age can end up feeling like their changing body is unattractive, which can lead them to eat more, in the hope that they will become less "desirable". And people who have been deprived of food as children can end up having a fear of being hungry and therefore overcompensate as adults. That's why compassion and empathy are key.

"Simply prescribing therapy or dieting as a solution does not address the root causes of these challenges and can even exacerbate them," Dr Wolrich adds. "That's why it's crucial to approach the conversation about body size and health with an understanding of the complexities, and to prioritise the wellbeing and autonomy of individuals, rather than imposing societal expectations or stereotypes."

THE IMPACT OF WEIGHT STIGMA ON HEALTH

As mentioned back in Chapter 2, *weight stigma* can, incredibly, have *more* of an impact on our health than actual increased *weight*. Dr Wolrich says on this matter: "In technical terms, the amount of allostatic load* caused by the stress and stigma of constantly having to justify one's appearance and perceived health to others, as well as self-judgement, can be overwhelming. The mere fact of constantly having to judge oneself and feeling like we've failed or not tried hard enough already puts a person at a disadvantage in life. ... it's unrealistic to believe that this level of stress and pressure won't have a negative impact on health."

---

* Allostatic load refers to the damage chronic stress can do to our bodies over time. It's the way stress and other things that affect our physical health can add up and cause problems like heart disease, diabetes and depression. Basically, it's the overall wear and tear that stress puts on all the different parts of our body.

Recent studies have even shown that the impact of weight stigma on health is comparable to that of racism. "However, where the comparisons stop," notes Dr Wolrich, "is that while we're happy to say things like 'just lose weight, then' to people in bigger bodies, we would never suggest an end to racism by saying 'Have you tried not being black?'"

"The root causes of racism and body size are," he says, "complex and intertwined with other factors, such as access to healthcare, exposure to stress and discrimination and genetics." This reinforces the fact that the right approach is never to tell someone to "just lose weight" or "just go to therapy", but instead to address the complex root causes of the issues and work towards creating a more inclusive and equitable society.

WHY BMI IS BOLLOCKS

Doctors tend to rely a lot on what is known as our BMI, or body mass index, to decide if we're "healthy" or not. BMI is calculated by dividing our weight in kilograms by our height in meters squared. And the resulting number puts us in the category of "underweight", "healthy", "overweight" or "obese".

The main reason I don't like BMI is because it's flawed (read on for more on this), but I also really dislike the "labels" that it gives people. I mean, what do the terms "underweight" and "overweight" really mean? ("Under" or "over" *what* weight?) And why is a term like "obese", which has been overwhelmingly used to insult and discriminate, being used in the context of defining our health?

You might find it interesting to know that, before BMI, the concept of "normal weight" was introduced in the early 1900s by health insurance companies, which had become increasingly popular in North America. Analysts had realised that policy holders with a greater weight-to-height ratio had the greatest mortality risk, so they introduced something called the "Metropolitan Life" tables. These tables were used by the companies to figure out how long someone might live and how much should therefore be charged for their insurance based on their age, gender and life expectancy, among other factors. At the time, the Metropolitan Life tables were seen as very important. However, there were a few major flaws, in that all the participants were white and it was assumed that men lived longer than women. Astoundingly, the tables were used by insurance companies up until as recently as 1985, when they were finally replaced. And this is where BMI enters the chat.

The truth about BMI is that it was never intended to measure health at an individual level, but at a population level. Even its inventor, Belgian statistician Adolphe Quetelet, outlined its flaws for measuring health way back in the 19th century. Quetelet knew that BMI wouldn't take into account certain important factors, given that he had originally come up with the idea to study health trends in groups of people, not to assess an individual's health. Below are just a couple of the issues that make BMI a flawed benchmark for overall health:

"Overweight" is not a synonym for "unhealthy"

Higher BMI is correlated with certain conditions on a population level, such as hypertension and cardiovascular disease, but there is actually very little evidence that higher weights cause these in *individuals*.

Nevertheless, as a result of so much emphasis in Western culture on BMI and thinness, things can get oversimplified, which means that people with high BMIs are sometimes denied certain care and treatments (such as IVF or surgeries), and weight loss is often presented as a cure-all.

Consider a patient with knee pain: if the person is *not* fat, they're likely to receive scans and treatment for the knee pain at the time of the complaint. If the person *is* fat, however, the doctor might diagnose *weight* as the problem, prescribe weight loss as the treatment and send them on their way without further diagnostic tests or treatments. In handling things this way for the fat person, not only might the doctor miss a problem that would have been visible on an X-ray or other imaging, but also the way the patient has been dealt with may well discourage bigger people from seeking any medical care at all about *other* things, therefore possibly worsening health issues.

In truth, you can be heavy and healthy, just as you can be thin and unhealthy. Researchers estimate that nearly 75 million adults in the US have their health misclassified on the basis of BMI, meaning that conditions have been missed or mistreated, wrong diagnoses given and incorrect treatments undertaken (*International Journal of Obesity,* 2016).

What's more, a study published in the *Journal of the American Medical Association* in 2013 looked at data from over 2.8 million adults and found that people with a BMI between 25 and 30 (the "overweight" category) had a lower mortality risk than people with a BMI between 18.5 and 25 (the "healthy" category).

Another study published in the *International Journal of Epidemiology* in 2015 looked at data from over 4 million adults and found that people who were classified as "overweight" or "obese" based on their BMI had the same mortality risk as people who were classified as "healthy". The study found that the lowest mortality risk was actually in the "overweight" category, while the highest mortality risk was in the "underweight" category.

BMI doesn't take into account race, ethnicity or body shape

BMI is calculated based on a person's weight and height, without taking into account their body composition. This means that people with a high proportion of muscle mass, such as athletes, can be classified as overweight or obese based on their BMI, despite having a low percentage of body fat. Meanwhile, someone with a low BMI might still have too much body fat and be at risk of health problems.

It also ignores differences in body shape and fat distribution, which can impact a person's health risks. For example, research suggests that people who carry more fat around their waist have a higher risk of heart disease and other health problems than those who carry fat in other parts of their body.

While BMI is calculated the same way for everyone, research shows that a person's BMI means different things for different ethnic groups. Among the white population, for example, the chances of issues associated with metabolic syndromes such as diabetes and heart disease go up at a BMI of 30, whereas in people of Indian descent, this happens at a BMI of 27, and the threshold for people of Taiwanese descent is even lower.

Other research has shown that the BMI associated with people who live longest is around 23 to 25 for white people, but 23 to 30 for black people, which means that a higher BMI could be beneficial for some black people. While weight stigma and inadequate care are bad for all, misclassifying black people as "overweight" may add to an already wide racial health disparity.

WHY DO WE CONTINUE TO USE BMI IF IT'S FLAWED?

The answer is simple (and incredibly frustrating): we don't yet have anything better that can provide the level of detail and accuracy needed to more accurately assess health.

BMI is easy to calculate and cheap to measure, and it's the basis of decades of health research. It's also deeply entrenched in the healthcare system. For example, in the US, BMI is embedded into the coding system that doctors use to let insurance companies know what they're billing for. And in the UK, it's used as a screening tool for everything from surgery to fertility treatment.

As I mentioned back in Chapter 1, after a couple of years of trying for a baby, my husband and I sought medical help. During our first appointment (after having been on a waiting list for nearly 10 months to *get* said appointment!), we were told, quite abruptly, that even investigative tests couldn't be carried out because of our high BMI. Yet, years later, after saving up enough money for private tests and treatment, we discovered that our infertility had absolutely nothing to do with our weight. Pretty disgraceful, really. So it would be great if healthcare providers could move beyond weight-based assumptions and discrimination, and instead prioritise comprehensive and unbiased assessments of an individual's health and needs. This shift would not only promote accurate diagnoses, but also ensure that every patient receives fair and equitable care, irrespective of their body size or appearance.

"IT'S BECAUSE YOU'RE FAT"

Look, let's be honest: doctors are highly educated people and I respect how hard their job is, but, as I mentioned earlier, they're subject to the same biases as the rest of us. I can't tell you how many times I've gone to the doctors for something as simple as an ear infection and been told to lose weight. And I'm by no means alone in this.

Here are just some of the things women I surveyed told me they'd experienced when going to see their doctor:

- "I have a family history of skin cancer and went to see my doctor about an unusual mole. He told me my weight wasn't helping."
- "I was diagnosed with depression and told that if I lost weight, it would magically go away."
- "I wasn't able to walk on my foot for months and was told it was because of my weight. But, after months of agony, I got a second opinion and found out I had a break."
- "I went to get a repeat prescription for my contraceptive pill and was told obese people like me cost the NHS millions."
- "I was struggling with anxiety and stress after working as a nurse on the frontline during Covid, and was told to lose weight."
- "I have problems with my knee and was told to lose 2 stone (28 lb/13 kg) before they would even do a scan."
- "I have lupus and my weight is ALWAYS mentioned when I go to the doctor's. It really puts me off going."
- "When I was pregnant, I was told I would probably miscarry because of my weight."

It's clear from these stories alone that the medical profession needs to step up. It needs to accept that fatness isn't the universal cause of ill health in fat people. It needs to accept that diets aren't the universal treatment option for fat people. And it needs to engage not only with the very real damage being caused by its prejudiced attitudes towards fat people, but also with the sub-standard care that's being delivered to many people as a result of their size.

Claire, 49, from Blackpool, England, went to see her doctor in 2016 for a suspected chest infection. She was told that she was grossly overweight and would end up "bankrupting" the NHS if she didn't do something to help herself. Because of that experience, she didn't see her doctor again for years. In 2022, she was struggling with severe pain in her abdomen as well as numerous other debilitating symptoms, but was too afraid to seek medical help. She died of ovarian cancer three months later.

So I'm not exaggerating when I say that lives actually *depend* on things drastically changing within the healthcare system when it comes to how doctors handle the relationship between weight and health.

WHAT'S THE SOLUTION?

While weight has been a prominent topic in medical training and education for years, I learned from speaking with Dr Wolrich that this training often promotes what is known as a "weight-normative" approach to healthcare – an approach that puts the emphasis on weight and weight loss when defining health and wellbeing.

Dr Wolrich believes that this weight-normative approach urgently needs to be re-evaluated, and that medical professionals should be trained to avoid harmful and stigmatising practices related to weight management: "Health should be the focus, not weight," he says, "and patients deserve to receive evidence-based recommendations and support in achieving their health goals." This would all be part of what is known as a "weight-inclusive" approach.

It seems that a lot of medical professionals could also do with better training in nutritional science, given that many of them have been shown to rely on their own experiences when it comes to discussing weight loss with their patients. Dr Wolrich rightly points out that this can then lead to "a spread of misinformation and non-evidence-based recommendations".

He goes on to say that the approach to weight should not be the same as the approach to other health risks. For example, even though height has been linked to a higher risk of cancer, nobody suggests stunting growth or preventing children from growing taller as a solution. The same should therefore be true for weight – a *range* of body sizes should be considered normal and healthy, without trying to impose a one-size-fits-all solution.

In summary, if obesity really is as major a health concern as the term "obesity epidemic" would imply, doctors need to start looking at the overall picture of every person's health, not just the size of their body if they happen to be fat. "To truly promote healthy behaviours, we need to move away from focusing on weight loss and instead focus on the inherent benefits and value of nutrition, exercise and sleep, while acknowledging the harms of stress, stigma and discrimination," says Dr Wolrich. "I would rather we just stop focusing on weight, full stop."

A NEW APPROACH:
THE HEALTH AT EVERY SIZE MOVEMENT

Now that you know just how inaccurate a measure of true health BMI is (at least in my humble opinion), and how much "healthier" a weight-inclusive approach to health would be (rather than a weight-normative one), you might be pleased to know about a new(ish) movement called Health at Every Size (HAES), which gained momentum in the 1990s. It supports ending weight discrimination, promotes health equity, seeks to downplay weight loss as a health goal and seeks to improve access to quality healthcare regardless of size.

HAES has three main components:

1. Acknowledging the impact of weight stigma and discrimination

HAES notes just how damaging an effect weight stigma and discrimination can have on our health – something that it's crucial for us all to start talking about more.

2. Healthcare beyond weight

HAES notes that weight is just one of *many* factors that contribute to our health, rather than the sole or main factor.

3. Weight-inclusive care

As the name of the HAES approach implies, it focuses on "health at every size". This weight-inclusive approach recognises that weight can sometimes change as a by-product of health-promoting behaviours, such as regular exercise, and that this change isn't the sole indicator of improved health.

Note that there's a big difference between the concepts of "Healthy at Every Size" (HAES) and "healthy at *any* size". HAES is not necessarily saying that every person can be healthy at any size. Instead, its aim is to shift the conversation to prioritise overall health (rather than weight) for *all* people of *all* sizes. For more information on HAES, read *Health at Every Size* by Linda Bacon (2010).

IS IT EVER OK TO WANT TO LOSE WEIGHT?

Weight loss is, of course, an individual choice. But I believe that, before we ever embark on any intentional weight loss, the most important thing is to look at *why* we want to lose weight. Is it for medical (and therefore health) reasons, like having surgery? Or is it, ultimately, just because we'd like to be thinner, and therefore conform to society's norms about what's more attractive (even if we're telling ourselves it's for "health reasons")?

Dr Wolrich says about this: "If you express a desire to lose weight because you don't feel healthy, the first thing I'd ask is why you believe losing weight will lead to improved health. The objective shouldn't be solely focused on changing the number on the scale; it should be about enhancing our overall wellbeing."

If we're focused solely on losing weight and obsessing over every pound that we do (or don't) lose, it can be demotivating and lead to behaviours such as crash dieting and excessive exercise, which aren't sustainable. If, on the other hand, we focus on improving our *overall* health, we're more likely to make lifestyle changes that can benefit our wellbeing in the long run, such as implementing a balanced and nutritious diet, engaging in regular, moderate exercise that we enjoy, getting adequate sleep, reducing stress levels and practising self-care.

While the temptation is strong to want to lose weight just in order to feel more accepted, etc., we have to weigh up the costs. "Is the continuous cycle of dieting and calorie counting worth it?" asks Dr Wolrich. "Frequently, the answer is no. As even when we reach our lowest weight, are we genuinely content? Again, the answer is usually no."

Think about this. Have you ever looked back at old photos of yourself, when you were in a smaller body, and thought "God, I wish I looked like that now!"? I know I have! Yet I can also remember that, at the time, I hated my body and how I looked, which is proof that it's never been about being a specific weight or size.

The hard truth is that, often, even if we *do* reach a target weight, it doesn't guarantee happiness. But making peace with the idea that the weight-loss goal you had set for yourself may not bring the happiness you were expecting is tough. Research shows that it can feel like a loss, and could even trigger a grieving process. "But once we acknowledge this truth," says Dr Wolrich, "we can start to focus on what truly matters – on what will improve our health, rather than what society thinks of us."

Studies have shown that there are many other aspects of health that are just as, if not more, important than weight. These can include factors such as improved energy levels, better digestion, and improved mental health. So, while it is, of course, OK to focus on losing weight if you really *want* to, it's likely to be more effective if you focus on making all-round healthy lifestyle changes as part of your journey of growth and self-discovery throughout life, rather than always feeling that you *have* to be on a diet.

WHAT DOES HEALTH MEAN TO YOU?

When I was younger, I definitely associated health with a particular aesthetic. For me, this meant being thinner, more toned, more ripped, more athletic and eating nothing but "clean" foods. I now understand that it's so much more than just these bodily aspects, of course.

I guess I've got to a "sweet spot" on my own personal journey with body image and health, where I feel comfortable in my skin (most of the time),

I don't let my weight hold me back and I want to fully accept myself as I am, yet I want to make all-round healthier lifestyle choices, too.

And I want you to be able to find your own unique "sweet spot" when it comes to your own relationship with both your weight and your health. So, remember:

- Health is NOT just about weight; it's about all sorts of things like levels of movement, nutrition, sleep, stress and much more.
- Be sure to advocate for yourself, if required, when you see any medical professional – ideally by calling them out on any anti-fat bias that you experience, or, otherwise, by switching health provider.
- You can, and should, live your life to the full in the body you have now, instead of fruitlessly waiting to be a smaller size.
- Even if you aren't healthy right now, you are still deserving of dignity and respect.

SELF-EMPOWERMENT TASK

Take a little time out for yourself and think of some things that you could do to improve your overall physical and/or mental health without referencing your size or weight loss.

This might include, for example, things like finding, and regularly doing, a form of exercise that you love and that makes you feel good, or nourishing your body with a variety of nutrient-rich foods including fruits, vegetables, whole grains, lean proteins and healthy fats so you feel more energised.

Feel free to write down anything that you think might particularly help you move forward in terms of your overall health, and therefore help you "take back the power" over your own body image, which is what we'll be discussing in Part 2.

PART 2

TAKING BACK THE POWER

Now you've finished Part One, how are you feeling? It's a lot to take in, I know.

But hopefully you can start to see just how much the odds have been stacked against us – and how we've been manipulated for SO long – by the media, by diet culture and by beauty standards – to feel like we're not good enough.

We never really stood a chance, did we?

What we're going to do next is take that frustration and use it to unlearn some of the BS we've been taught over the years.

It's time to take back the power …

7

Body positivity or body neutrality?
What should I be aiming for?

I want to start this part of the book by talking about the body positivity movement. More specifically, I want to delve into where it started, what it was *meant* to be and what it has become now. Why? Because there are so many misconceptions about what being "body positive" actually means.

Lots of people think that body positivity *literally* means that you have to feel positive about your body all the time, while others seem to believe that it means you have free rein to eat 40 pizzas and 10 tubs of ice cream a day (spoiler alert: it doesn't).

What a lot of people don't know is that before the body positivity movement, there was the Fat Acceptance Movement. The fight for fat acceptance first gained traction in the 1960s, as more and more people began to recognise the rampant discrimination and stigma fat people were facing in their daily lives.

"The Fat Acceptance Movement was built on a foundation laid by fat, black, queer women in the civil rights and welfare rights movements, and was centred on the fair treatment of fat people," explains Stephanie Yeboah, blogger, body-image advocate and author of *Fattily Ever After*. The movement was deeply significant because, as Yeboah says, "The black female body has been dehumanised, mammified, hypersexualised and fetishised since the days of slavery, by the patriarchy and by white society."

One of the most visible early actions of the movement was a "fat-in" held in New York City in 1967. This event drew hundreds of protesters determined to challenge the prevailing narrative about fatness and obesity. They burned diet books, carried signs declaring "Fat Power" and called for equal treatment for everyone, regardless of body size, as well as an end to anti-fat discrimination. *The New York Times* covered the event, giving it the headline "Curves Have Their Day in Park: 500 at a 'Fat-in' Call for Obesity". Disappointingly (although not surprisingly), the article failed to recognise the seriousness of the protestors' demands, instead insinuating they were "promoting obesity" and other unhealthy behaviours. Some things never change, eh?

Just one year later, the National Association to Advance Fat Acceptance (NAAFA) was founded in the US by two men called Lew Louderback and Bill Fabrey. Both were married to fat women and had witnessed first-hand the biased and discriminatory treatment that their wives (and other fat individuals) endured. NAAFA quickly became a key organisation in the fight for fat acceptance, advocating for better representation in media and employment protections, as well as improved access to healthcare.

One of the criticisms of the movement at the time was that it often ignored the voices of people of colour, with some white activists arguing that taking on more than one issue at a time (i.e. racism as well as fat-ism) might dilute their message. Some also believed that black communities and other communities of colour were already more accepting of fat people, leading them to believe that fat activism wasn't needed in those areas.

Because of this, a group of feminists based in California formed their own alliance called the Fat Underground. While NAAFA championed fat acceptance, the Fat Underground fought for fat liberation, releasing a seminal manifesto in 1973 that demanded equal rights for fat people in all areas of life.

While the Fat Acceptance Movement focused on promoting acceptance and respect for people of all sizes, the Fat Underground, motivated by the leadership they saw in the civil rights movement, went further by seeking to dismantle the systems of oppression and discrimination faced by fat people, as well as other women in marginalised bodies: black women, disabled women, and queer women.

The Fat Underground wasn't just a group of individuals advocating for body positivity; it was a political movement that aimed to change the way society viewed and treated fat people. They argued that discrimination against fat people was a form of oppression rooted in capitalism, patriarchy and white supremacy. The movement was sparked in part by the book *Fat is a Feminist Issue*, by Susie Orbach, which challenged the notion that thinness was the ideal female body type. This book, along with other feminist writings of the time, really paved the way for a wider conversation about body size and discrimination.

The aim of the Fat Underground was to change the narrative of fatness as a personal flaw to fatness as a societal issue, with the philosophy of "change society, not ourselves" serving as the foundation. Despite some setbacks, the movement continued to gain momentum and, by the mid-1980s, the enthusiasm had spread as far as the UK, leading to the formation of the London Fat Women's Group.

However, the move from underground to mainstream took somewhat longer, as it really wasn't until the early 2000s that "body positivity" became a buzzword on people's lips, with brands even starting to incorporate it into their marketing …

THE DARKER SIDE OF BODY POSITIVITY

The cultural evolution of body positivity entered its next chapter in 2011, when it began appearing in newly popular plus-sized fashion blogs. As the decade progressed, early blogging platforms such as LiveJournal became obsolete and were replaced by an abundance of microblogging sites like Tumblr. Because of this, the once-niche fat-positive movement gave way to a much looser interpretation of body positivity. And that's when things started to get somewhat messy.

By the time I came across the body positivity movement (around 2018), it was a somewhat diverse, social-media-based community celebrating self-love and radical self-acceptance of fat bodies of all races. But not long after that, the movement started to become heavily commodified by mainstream culture and commercial interests.

One common criticism is that the movement became watered down and depoliticised, with its original message of challenging oppressive beauty standards and promoting radical self-love being replaced by a more superficial message of "loving your flaws" and promoting self-confidence. This led to a focus on individual people and their appearance, rather than on systemic issues such as fatphobia, racism and ableism.

In Yeboah's view, the introduction of the concept "all bodies matter" glossed over the abuse, marginalisation and "othering" of unprivileged bodies that had always fallen outside the scope of what was seen as "beautiful". And so, it made the movement into one that aimed to remove the prejudices that make us value some bodies more than others.

"It is incredibly political, something that should not be overlooked or forgotten," she says. "And like feminism, any approach to body positivity that refuses to acknowledge hierarchies of privilege – that refuses to learn from those who are more oppressed, and that neglects to fight for those more marginalised – is missing something crucial."

And it's fair to say that, since the 1990s, the movement has pretty much been dominated by white, straight, able-bodied and conventionally "attractive" people, which has meant a lack of representation for people of colour (especially darker-skinned black women), disabled people and others who don't fit within conventional beauty ideals, i.e. the very people who established the concept in the first place!

The commercialisation of the body positivity movement continued – with, as briefly mentioned, many brands and influencers now using it as a marketing tool to sell products – and with it came accusations of "woke-washing" (i.e. brands flashing support for just causes without demonstrating any real commitment to the values) and of social-justice language being used to promote consumerism, diluting the movement's original message and erasing its radical roots.

Seeing fat, black women in the media, owning their confidence and sexuality, has always been an extreme rarity. And this sparse representation is not enough. While the body positivity movement has undoubtedly made progress in terms of promoting inclusivity, it has also created its own set of standards that can be harmful to individuals who already face marginalisation or underprivilege.

It seems to me that the focus has shifted from celebrating plus-size women and challenging traditional beauty standards to promoting a new beauty ideal that excludes more people than not. This new ideal instead centres on women who are deemed "acceptable fat", i.e. women smaller than a UK size 16 (US size 12), who often have hourglass figures, are conventionally pretty and typically of a light-skinned complexion.

Some such women can be found on social media distorting their bodies to create rolls and folds when, in reality, there are none. They are the same type of women who tell us that it's OK to gain weight or go up a jeans size, while using the hashtag #bodypositivity or #BoPo – when, in reality, lots of us would be sized out of mainstream clothing if we did so (if we aren't already).

Personally, I just don't think that the recent focus within the movement on the need to love ourselves and embrace every aspect of our bodies is realistic. And while the "all bodies are beautiful" message that body positivity has become synonymous with is a step in the right direction, it seems, to me, to incorrectly reinforce the core belief that looking good and feeling beautiful is a prerequisite to happiness.

It's for this reason, as well as the white-washing, that lots of people who previously championed the body positivity movement now don't want to be associated with it, as they feel it no longer reflects them or their values.

One of those people is Yeboah. She says: "Once a movement hits the mainstream, it runs the risk of being diluted – or worse, capitalised upon – and that's exactly what happened to body positivity. As soon as the movement picked up steam, it took on a secondary messaging that "all bodies are beautiful", and was then hijacked by people who fall within what society considers beautiful (white and thin). It's incredibly frustrating."

Because body positivity has now been depoliticised, Yeboah and others have shifted back to using terms like "fat liberation" and "fat acceptance" – bringing the movement back to what it was in the first place. What's so disheartening, though, is that these terms are rarely, if ever, used by people who claim to be "body positive". When it's not as buzzword-y, trendy or profitable (and because it includes the word "fat"), there's little interest. And suddenly, the body positivity movement feels a bit bleak.

This is where body neutrality enters the chat.

THE RISE OF BODY NEUTRALITY

Because of how much the body positivity movement has spilled over into our mainstream culture, I get asked by women all the time: "How do I love my body?" But I'm going to let you in on a secret: you don't have to.

For too long we've been sold this lie that we have to be "body positive", love every inch of ourselves and embrace our "flaws". But it's just not true. I don't love my stomach, or the pigmentation under my armpits, or my upper thighs, and I don't think it's realistic for me to love myself every single day.

For me, it's about accepting all these things and getting on with my life regardless.

I know my worth doesn't lie in my appearance, and I know the way I look is the least interesting thing about me. And *that's* the beauty of the body-neutrality movement.

What exactly is body neutrality?

Body neutrality centres on basic RESPECT and ACCEPTANCE for your body over all-out love. In a nutshell, it:

- Removes guilt on the more difficult body-image days
- Provides a middle ground between the moments you love your body and the moments when you may dislike it
- Prioritises what makes your body work/feel good/function best over constant thoughts about losing weight, what you see in the mirror and/or how you look
- Asks questions like "What does this body part help me do?", "Is there anything that is good that comes from it?" and "Is there space to respect, value, or honour my body in any way?"
- Challenges you to think about your body as something you care about
- Challenges you to think about where any thoughts of negativity about your body come from

While the concept of body neutrality has been around for a while, it really only gained traction in the early 2010s.

One of the earliest advocates of the movement was Kelsey Miller, a journalist and author who chronicled her journey towards body acceptance in her memoir, *Big Girl*. In the book, Miller writes about her experiences with body positivity and how it ultimately left her feeling like a failure when she was unable to fully embrace her body as beautiful.

Miller's story resonated with a lot of women who had struggled with body positivity and were looking for an alternative. Soon, other advocates began to emerge, sharing their own stories and promoting the idea of body neutrality as a way to break free from the cycle of body shame and self-hatred.

The concept of body neutrality is simple: instead of placing a value judgement on our bodies, it encourages us to accept them – just as they are – without expectation. The philosophy is basically "I have a body, and so does everyone else". As such, it's essentially about focusing on how your body feels and what it can do for you, instead of what it looks like. This means recognising your body's value beyond its appearance, instead cultivating a sense of gratitude for its capabilities, whether that's enabling you to move, breathe, experience the world around you or whatever else.

Clinical psychologist Dr Emma Cotterill says focusing on what your body *can* do is absolutely crucial for us to quieten the "noise" around our appearance. "This might be recognising that our body is able: to move, to get to work, to carry a baby, to hold a partner's hand, to have sex, to engage in a hobby, to reach a goal or to spend time with friends," she says. "Really think about all the amazing things your body can do, or has done over the years. And gently acknowledge any challenges it has faced – if you've experienced illness, or health problems, or injuries. Remind yourself that this is the only body you'll ever have, and to be on your own team."

In practical terms, body neutrality might also involve tuning into your body's needs and desires, such as eating when you're hungry and stopping eating when you're full, regardless of what the scale or societal norms might dictate.

Another key aspect of body neutrality is letting go of the constant self-criticism and negative self-talk that can be so damaging to our mental health. Instead of obsessing over perceived flaws or imperfections, body neutrality encourages us to simply observe our bodies with curiosity.

One early advocate of body neutrality was Jameela Jamil, actress and founder of social justice movement iWeigh. She said in a 2019 interview with *Glamour* magazine: "Imagine just not thinking about your body. You're not hating it. You're not loving it. You're just a floating head. I'm a floating head wandering through the world."

BODY-NEUTRAL AFFIRMATIONS

1. I am more than just my appearance

2. My worth doesn't depend on how I look or how much I weigh

3. It's OK for my body image to change

4. I don't need to feel attractive to enjoy my life and relationships

5. I accept my body as it is right now

6. I appreciate my body and what it does for me

7. My body works hard and deserves compassion

8. My relationship with my body is no one's business but my own

9. I deserve to nourish myself with food

10. My body is the least interesting thing about me

WHAT'S WRONG WITH DERIVING CONFIDENCE FROM THE WAY YOU LOOK?

There's nothing wrong with deriving some confidence from the way you look. But I do think it's important that we avoid basing our entire self-worth on it.

It's inevitable that our bodies will change throughout our lifetime, whether it's through pregnancy, illness, hormonal changes, weight loss, weight gain or just ageing. So, if we've always relied on feeling attractive to feel good about ourselves, what happens if something about our appearance suddenly changes, such as drastic weight gain or a bout of acne? Chances are it could leave us in a tailspin.

"Feeling good about yourself is a basic human need," says psychotherapist, body-image specialist and mental health practitioner, Dr Holli Rubin. "The problem is that society has taught us the importance of being beautiful over anything else. And that's not a healthy mindset to have. Body neutrality is really powerful because it focuses on function over form."

So, while it's fine to care about what you look like and take pleasure from a snazzy haircut or nice new dress, just make sure you have other things in your life to fall back on that will contribute to your sense of self-worth and provide you with a deeper sense of purpose. Instead of focusing solely on what you look like, you might therefore want to start thinking about, for example, what skills, talents and strengths you have, what achievements you're most proud of, and what challenges you've overcome. This might feel odd, or tricky, at first if you're not used to it, but stick with it and it will gradually get easier with practice …

IS BODY NEUTRALITY RIGHT FOR ME?

Although body neutrality has many benefits, I think it's important to mention that it's more difficult for some people than others. The fact that body neutrality focuses on appreciation for specific things that the body can *do* means that it isn't inclusive of everyone.

Some members of the disabled community, for example, have spoken up about the ableism associated with the body-neutral approach, given that it focuses on body functioning, which can differ considerably from person to person. They make a very good point that your body's ability to do certain things for you should not determine your body image or self-esteem, especially since our body's capacities can change over time for various reasons.

Below are the stories of two women who I spoke to about their struggle with body neutrality:

Body neutrality is great in the fact that it allows us to understand ourselves and others on a deeper level, to value us internally as well as externally. It does seem like a much more balanced approach to life but it can also be difficult for me to be body neutral because of my disability. My body sometimes lets me down; I get fatigue and I get frustrated when I can't do certain things. It can be hard to detach myself from this! I don't think disabled people like myself will ever be able to be fully "body neutral" until we see more people like us on a global scale – in magazines, in advertising, in mainstream media – but also until we are able to do simple things like leave the house and not worry about access. Bigger changes need to happen where we are fully accepted in society, and only then can we start to live comfortably in our bodies.
– Sophie

"Neutrality", to me, suggests the goal is to emotionally detach from our body – refuse to tie our identity to any aspect of our appearance. At best, this goal would be leave us indifferent towards our bodies. At worst, it implies our bodies play no role in forming our sense of self.

Neither of these outcomes seems attainable, at least to me, as a big, bald, blotchy woman … I started losing my hair aged just 13, just as hormones were flying about and we were all – literally – sizing each other up. Now, nearly two decades after discovering and swiftly hiding that first bald patch, I'm finally accepting my alopecia.

But I'm not just learning to "accept" my body, I am actively attempting to unlearn all that society has taught me about my value as someone with visible difference. I am not "indifferent" or "neutral", about this, I'm passionate. In fact, I may even be angry. Angry that I ever felt lesser for being overweight; ashamed that I ever felt being bald meant I was unloveable; and upset that I wore a wig that left my head with open sores, rather than consider simply existing without it.

I am no longer prioritising society's comfort at the expense of my body's discomfort. My relationship with my body is far from "neutral", and I don't want it to be. I want to acknowledge the unhealthy obsession that I, and we all, seem to have with what bodies look like. My goal is instead to transform the energy I've wasted hiding my "flaws" into something positive. My bald head is becoming a huge part of my identity as a powerful campaigner and I am going to lean into that now, and for the rest of my life.
– Laura M

BODY NEUTRALITY AS THE FOUNDATION FOR SELF-ACCEPTANCE?

While the concept of body neutrality obviously has its limitations for some people, discovering it allowed me to acknowledge the fraught relationship that I had up until that point with my body. Previously, I'd been *saying* that I loved it, but, in reality, that was only on very rare occasions. So, for me, admitting that I would possibly never really *love* my body felt like a big step towards freeing my self-worth from what I look like.

My hope is that leaning into body neutrality might help you in some similar way.

By the way, despite having come a long way on my body-neutrality journey, I still have bad body-image days. And I think these are inevitable. So please know that if you have these too, it doesn't mean you're getting anything wrong. You're just trying to unlearn a lifetime of body shame while still navigating toxic beauty standards everywhere you turn.

So remember: you're allowed to have bad days, you're allowed to miss your old, smaller body, you're allowed to be tempted by diets and diet culture …

But also remember: you deserve better than *only* that, so keep coming back to knowing that your body *isn't* the problem, to knowing that you're doing your best, and to knowing that your body is "enough" just as it is.

The reason I'm such a supporter of body neutrality is that I believe, for many, it can lay the foundation for self-acceptance, which is what we're going to delve into in the next chapter. But for now, I have another little "task" for you.

SELF-EMPOWERMENT TASK

Take a little time out for yourself and write down all the things that your body can do for you that have nothing to do with what you look like – everything from breathing and digesting food to seeing and hearing, walking and running, dancing and jumping.

You can get more specific, if you like, by including particular skills or hobbies that you have, or activities that you do.

There's no right or wrong here, as it's all about what YOU recognise and are grateful for when it comes to your own unique body …

8

The road to self-acceptance

Acknowledging your body for what it is - unique and imperfectly perfect

How many opportunities have you missed out on because of your body? I dread to think how much time and energy I've wasted over the years worrying about what I look like and what other people think of me.

My journey towards self-acceptance started after deciding not to have bariatric surgery in 2020. I still wanted to lose weight at that stage, but, for the first time in my life, I started to think about whether that was realistically on the cards for me, or whether it needed to be.

Not long after that came the Covid outbreak. Thoughts of "I could be dead tomorrow" swirled around my head and ignited a zest for life in me that I hadn't had before. I suddenly realised all the precious time that I had wasted hating myself and how I looked. Thoughts of "What diet am I going to do next to lose weight?" slowly turned into "Is it the worst thing in the world if I *don't* lose weight? and "What would happen if, maybe, I just tried accepting myself instead?"

I fought for a long time with the idea of accepting myself, because it felt like it would mean "giving up". I felt that's what other people would think, at least, and that they would judge me for it. But the rebellious side of me then started to take over, leading me, as mentioned in Chapter 1, to start doing a lot of research into the toxic world of diet culture; to start wearing colour (rather than black); to start buying clothes that actually fitted me (rather than waiting for Laura 2.0's new, smaller wardrobe); and to start travelling more too (even if it did mean needing a seatbelt extender).

I also started saying "no" more to things that I would have previously done only to please other people. And I started saying "yes" to activities that I wanted to do but normally wouldn't have done due to fear, such as the obstacle course on water that I completed a few years ago for my stepsister's hen do.

Thoughts of the wetsuit not going round me, or that I wouldn't be fit enough to complete the course, crippled me for months. But what crippled me more was the thought of being the person that stood on the side, just watching and taking pictures of everyone else getting stuck in, having a great time and making memories, like I used to. So, I got the damn wetsuit on, did the best I could on the course and, most importantly, I had fun!

Slowly but surely, I started to accept myself instead of hating myself, and I can honestly say it's the most life-changing thing I've ever done.

I don't love my body every day. I don't even like it most days. But I try and accept it and not beat myself up about it. Why? Because I've realised that life is too short, too precious, too fleeting to miss out on any more chances at happiness.

I don't want to waste my life worrying that I don't look like a Kardashian. And I don't want that for you, either. In this chapter, we'll therefore take an in-depth look at self-acceptance, and most importantly, how to do things that scare you, have fun and live life to the full, without letting your body hold you back in any way.

ACCEPTING YOUR BODY AS IT IS

As I see it, there are three main steps towards self-acceptance.

First, we need to shift our focus from "fixing" ourselves to accepting ourselves. Instead of trying to change things about our appearance, we need to *celebrate* what our bodies can do for us.

Second, we need to stop comparing ourselves to others (easier said than done, I know), and remind ourselves that everyone's body is different, and we all have our own unique journey to health and happiness.

Finally, we need to remember that change is a slow and rarely linear process, which certainly doesn't happen overnight. The idea that we can transform ourselves in a few weeks or months is not only unrealistic, but also harmful. It sets us up for failure and disappointment when we don't see the same dramatic results as the people so often depicted in "before and after" photos.

So now that we know what we need to do, let's delve a bit deeper into how to do it.

Learning to accept our bodies is a challenge for many of us. As women, we've been taught to hate ourselves and reject our body unless it appears "perfect", which has always been a shifting mirage because a) the "perfect" body depicted in traditional media doesn't exist (we all know by now that editing software, used in multiple subtle ways, can create images that don't reflect reality, and so are impossible to live up to), and b) the idea of what is socially desirable constantly *changes* – we only have to look at the changing ideal body shape over the decades that we saw in Chapter 3 to see this is true.

With this in mind, here are some principles for you to take on board in order to help you accept your body:

1. Know that EVERY body is unique and EVERY body has lumps, bumps, squidgy bits, wrinkly bits, soft bits and different-coloured bits. EVERY body is imperfectly perfect.
2. Know that the media ideals of a perfect body are not only unattainable but impossible. They do not exist.
3. Remember you cannot hate your body into being something different.
4. Remember that this is your one body, so you can choose to spend your time hating it, or you can learn to accept it and be grateful for it.
5. Know that learning to accept your body doesn't mean you have to love it (although it's great if this can be a work in progress); it just means that we make peace with it being the one that we have.
6. Know that when you learn to accept your body, you're more likely to begin being kinder to it and to feel better in yourself (in terms of both mood and wellbeing).

GETTING COMFORTABLE WITH THE MIRROR

Being OK with what we look like in the mirror plays a large part in the journey towards self-acceptance. But for many of us, the mirror can be a source of great frustration and anxiety. Even those of us who have never been diagnosed with an eating disorder or body dysmorphia (which entails you seeing something completely different to reality in the mirror) can have a tendency to overestimate our size. In fact, women have been shown to overestimate the width of their cheeks, thighs, waist and hips by an average of 25% (*Journal of Translational Medicine*, 2014).

In a 2019 study published by the *International Journal of Eating Disorders*, women were asked to digitally adjust a distorted image of their body to match their real body as closely as possible. A group of researchers came up with the eye-tracking experiment to figure out why women perceive their own bodies so much more negatively (and less clearly) than other people's bodies. The participants included women who had been diagnosed with an eating disorder as well as control subjects who hadn't.

Participants who suffered from an eating disorder looked at their own bodies in a very particular way: they kept their eyes fixed on the body parts they considered unattractive and pretty much ignored the rest of their body. Yet they did the exact opposite when it came to other people's bodies: they kept their gaze on what they would later label as attractive parts and glossed over the rest.

Psychologists believe the same attentional bias is what's behind women misperceiving the way their body looks. When women walk past a mirror, they tend to focus on the parts that they consider to be "flaws" rather than the parts that they like. Researchers believe that the reason we do this is actually pretty simple: because, as humans, we are programmed to pay attention to things that we have strong feelings about or consider a threat. And, in a culture that equates beauty with value and loveability, "flaws" pose a "threat".

The problem is, of course, that if you only ever pay attention to what you consider your least attractive or biggest body parts while ignoring the rest, your perception of these parts takes over the picture you have of your entire body, and you'll think you're less attractive overall, or bigger than you really are.

So what can be done about this? Here are three solutions:

- Very intentionally focus on the positives. So instead of fixating on the parts of your body that you *don't* like, try to focus on the parts that you *do* like. This will involve trying to take a metaphorical step back every time you're at a mirror, in order to see yourself as a whole, rather than straight away zooming in on your flaws.
- Talk more kindly to yourself, preferably while looking in the mirror. This is because a 2017 study by Italian researchers showed that people who looked in the mirror while saying compassionate things to themselves felt even better than those who didn't use a mirror while engaging in positive self-talk. They experienced more soothing and positive emotions, and their heart rate variability (which is a good sign of emotional and physical wellbeing) was much better.
- Shift conversations away from outer appearance as much as possible, towards inner qualities such as kindness, intelligence and humour; the more we can do this, the less power physical "flaws" will have over our perception of ourselves.

SELF-EMPOWERMENT TASK

Take a little time out for yourself and, either naked or in underwear, stand in front of a full-length mirror, trying not to suck anything in or manipulate your body in any way (I know it's hard). Then say to yourself: "I am learning to accept you. You are a wonderful, normal, flawed human body and you are enough, just as you are."

Keep saying this for as long as it takes you to feel at least vaguely comfortable with it, or maybe even until you start to feel and believe it.

TAKING UP SPACE IN A WORLD THAT WANTS TO SHRINK YOU

Have you ever noticed how, in *The Little Mermaid*, Ursula's final act was to make herself even bigger? Her presence alone causes the sea to swell and surge, as she effortlessly commands the waves to follow her every whim. Her commanding presence transforms her into a sorceress, a queen and a goddess.

This unapologetic portrayal of a fat body as a dominant force is not one that we see very often in the media (if at all). And it really got me thinking how, in many ways, the unapologetic fat body serves as a symbol of resistance.

One of the hardest lessons I have had to learn, and, if I'm being honest, am still learning, is around taking up space and being unapologetic about it. I've always been fat, and that's meant always feeling the need to apologise for being too big, too clumsy, too in the way.

And nowhere is this truer than on public transport, as hinted at in my discussion about flying (and how much I used to fear it) back in Chapter 2. As I said there, I know that it's many people's worst nightmare to end up sitting next to someone as big as me when they're travelling. But we can't help needing to get on the train, bus or plane. And we can't help that the seats are teeny-tiny, either.

Some of the most anxiety-inducing experiences of my life have been on, or leading up to, getting on an aeroplane. For years I actually didn't go on holiday because I was worried about fitting in the seat or being fat-shamed, or both.

I now go on holidays and enjoy them to the full (see the box on page 148 for top tips for flying when fat). But my old fear about "being too big" and "taking up too much space" reared its head on a recent holiday when I struggled every evening to fit my ass into the stupidly narrow restaurant chairs. Embarrassed, I didn't want anyone to know, so I asked for a table at the very end of the restaurant each night, and I then lowered my hips in one at a time so that they could sit (almost) comfortably under the tight constraints of the chair arms above it.

Instead of speaking up on the first night of my holiday and risking "making a spectacle of myself", I tried to forget about it. But by night four I was starting to dread meal times, as I was actually in pain. So, I finally advocated for myself by asking for another chair. This might sound like a small thing to some, but it was a really difficult thing for me to do. Our holiday resort was full of what looked like Russian supermodels, and I felt like Shrek. But I asked for another chair, I got it, and no one died. Hurrah!

Here are some tips to help you advocate for yourself:

1. **Speak up:** Your voice matters, and you have the right to express your thoughts and opinions. So don't be afraid to make yourself heard, even if you feel like your ideas are different from others'.
2. **Stand tall:** Your body language can convey confidence and strength. So stand proud, with your shoulders back, head held high and feet planted firmly on the ground.
3. **Set boundaries:** It's OK to say no and put boundaries in place with people who may try to minimise your presence or take advantage of your kindness. Your time and energy are valuable, so make sure you prioritise your needs.
4. **Pursue your passions:** Don't let your body hold you back from doing what brings you joy and fulfilment, whether this is

creative pursuits, physical activity, travelling or volunteering in your local community. It's time to embrace and pursue your specific interests and talents, whatever they may be.

Another big lesson I've learned as part of advocating for myself in recent years is that I'm not actually the extrovert I thought I was; I'm actually quite shy and find social situations a bit anxiety-inducing. I've realised that my "bubbly" behaviour over the years was actually often me overcompensating for how I felt about my body – so that people thought I was at least a fun and nice person, "even though" I was fat.

Does any of this resonate with you? Are there ways that you behave in order to compensate for your appearance rather than because it feels like a true part of your personality? If so, it's time to let them go.

Remember, giving yourself permission to "take up space" is not about being loud, lively, bubbly or dominating; it's about simply asserting your right to exist and be seen. You are worthy of taking up space and living your best life, just as you are.

So please: book the holiday, take the trip, go to that place you've always dreamt of, be in the photos and make those memories. Life is for living.

TOP TIPS FOR FLYING WHEN FAT

Squeezing through the aisles with your bags, that uncomfortable feeling of needing to ask for a seatbelt extender, the annoyance of those around you – there's a whole lot to navigate when flying as a bigger-bodied person.

But here are some tips that I've picked up over the years to help get you through it, as much as can be anticipated:

- First, do your research on the different airlines and their seat widths, as they do vary. On easyJet, for example, the arm rest on most of the window seats go all the way up – giving you a little more space. Southwest Airlines offers a "Customer of Size" policy, which allows you to purchase the seat next to you to allow for extra room and then be refunded for the price of it post-flight. Those unable to afford doing so can arrive at the airport a few hours early and ask to utilise the policy; if there's space on the aircraft, they will enact the policy free of charge for you.

- When you board the plane, ask one of the flight attendants if you can move to a seat that has an empty one next to it. Plus-size travel expert Kirsty Leanne says this works for her 99% of the time.

- Don't be afraid to ask for a seatbelt extender. Why they make them bright orange is beyond me, but hey, safety comes first. You can ask for one before boarding the aircraft if you prefer. Any flight attendant worth their salt will hand it to you discreetly and professionally. You can also buy seatbelt extenders online beforehand (I have in the past and it massively helped reduce anxiety). I will say, however, that these aren't officially permitted by most airlines, so if they see it, they may ask you to use theirs.

- Ask for priority boarding if you can. Doing so will allow you to get comfortable and receive a seatbelt extender without the worry of having to squeeze past other passengers.

- Upgrade to premium economy or business class if you can afford it and/or want to. You'll get a lot more room and, generally speaking, the seatbelts are a bit longer.

- Don't book an "XL" seat or emergency row seat. An XL seat usually just means one with extra leg room and these are often in the emergency exit row. For safety reasons, you're not allowed to wear a seatbelt extender in these rows. I found this out the hard way during a trip to Tenerife, and was made to do the walk of shame, with my bright orange seatbelt extender, to a new seat just before take-off.

- Lastly, be vocal, even if it feels difficult to do so. For example, be upfront with the person you're sitting next to and tell them you won't be offended if they want to move. And if they're mean to you, please do speak up and tell a flight attendant. They should do everything they can to accommodate you.

Above all, remember you deserve to take up space and travel, just like everyone else.

NOT BEING THE "GOOD FATTY"

Because it's often implied that fat people are lazy, stupid and even unloveable, it's common for us to try to counteract this by being people-pleasers. As mentioned in Chapter 1, this is often why you find bigger people playing the role of the funny one, the "cuddly", caring one, the one that's great in the kitchen or whatever else – in order to mask their insecurities.

This is known in the fat-liberation movement as being a "good fatty". It's an expression that describes behaviours adopted to lessen the impact of stigma, and is often a coping mechanism for when that stigma is anticipated or felt.

Being a "good fatty" can mean telling everyone you're "being good" by ordering a salad, or something else low in calories at a restaurant, when you really want something else. It can mean standing on public transport so you don't take up two seats. It can mean wearing a cover-up on the beach for the sake of onlookers when you *really* want to wear a bikini. In doing such things, you're trying to make your fatness more "acceptable".

Growing up, I always felt the need to look as feminine as possible, with perfectly styled hair and the best clothes I could find in my size. It was as if I was trying to say: "See, I'm not a complete waste of space. I have highlights in my hair and I'm well put together!"

I got labelled "bubbly" (code for fat) a lot as a teenager, and I think that's because I tried to be everyone's friend. I would say what I thought everyone wanted to hear, instead of what I actually thought. I was always polite and asked questions. I was "little Miss Sunshine". I'm not sure who came up with the idea that fat people have to be jolly, but if there was a rule book on how to be a "good fatty", I'm pretty sure it would say: "It's bad enough that you're fat, god forbid, that you be fat and *miserable*. So smile more, please!"

Now that I'm in my 30s and know about this "good fatty" coping strategy, I'm more aware of when I'm doing it and I try to stop myself. That doesn't give me a pass to be a complete dick, of course; it just means never trying to be someone who I'm not. And this is a lot less exhausting than the alternative. While the habit takes a lot of unlearning, I think it's an important lesson for anyone in a marginalised body to learn.

So please remember your worth and check yourself the next time you go to make a joke at your own expense or go out of your way in any other way to try to make someone see that you're actually a pretty decent human being, not just a "fat bird". You really don't need the approval of others; all you need is your *own* approval.

SHIFTING THE FOCUS TO HEALTH INSTEAD OF APPEARANCE

Another key part of accepting ourselves and developing a psychologically healthier relationship with our bodies is widening the lens of what helps us to feel good in our body and mind to be more about our health – both physical and mental – instead of our appearance.

Clinical psychologist Dr Emma Cotterill says: "When we begin to take care of ourselves on a wider level, it creates a ripple effect which, ultimately, can positively affect how we feel about ourselves and our bodies." Her recommendations include:

- **Dealing with stressors head-on and watching out for burnout.** Stress affects our sleep, our mood, our eating and our relationships, so it's vital we manage it as best we can, share our stresses with others to alleviate them, write them down to help get them off our chest and problem-solve them, and seek support where we need.

- **Embarking on fun and meaningful hobbies.** Keeping active helps lift our mood, and doing things that we enjoy, are good at or gain a sense of achievement from helps improve both our confidence and motivation.

- **Maintaining social connections.** Spending time with others who we have a shared social connection with can boost mood, build our social confidence and soothe us, as it makes us feel included and part of a community.

- **Practising compassion over criticism, every day.** Learning ways to be more compassionate to ourselves in daily life has been proven to play a big part in our self-acceptance journey.

- **Practicing self-care and taking care of yourself and your body in little ways.** This could be taking time to sleep well, engaging in pampering activities, allowing yourself to rest, choosing clothes that fit you well, exercising for wellbeing and so on.

- **Practising focusing on health and wellbeing "success" for both yourself and others above weight or appearance "success".** Practise *not* commenting on others' weight loss, bodies or appearance. Instead, practise placing your focus on other positive attributes, qualities, interests and values. Practise encouraging your own success in making choices that benefit your health and wellbeing on a broader scale in all areas of your life.

HOW TO STOP COMPARING OURSELVES TO OTHERS

I had a friend growing up who I idolised. I wanted, more than anything, to be like her. She was the "cool kid" – the beautiful one with Bambi eyes, a great figure and amazing hair. All the boys worshipped her, and all the girls wanted to be her. I copied everything from her taste in music to her emo style.

One Saturday, I decided, in an attempt to be more like her, to dye my hair from bright blonde to jet black. My hairdresser warned me against it, my mum explicitly told me not to do it and even my friend thought it was a stupid idea. But for some reason, I'd clung onto this idea that this new hair colour would solve all my problems and make me prettier, better and more worthy. So, after much persuading, my hairdresser caved …

I'll never forget when she unwrapped the towel from my wet head. My heart sank and tears swelled in my eyes as I saw the mass of black hair against my pasty skin. I knew instantly that I'd made a terrible mistake (one that would take years – and a lot of money that I didn't have – to fix). And all because I was comparing myself to my "cool", naturally olive-skinned friend.

I look back and laugh now because I'm sure that was all normal teenage stuff, but I think it was deeper than that, too – it was a result of how I felt about my size. For most of my life, I've obsessed over other girls and women who were deemed beautiful, and tried to emulate what they had in order to feel better about myself, whether it be a hair colour (as in the case just described), a handbag or a new pair of shoes.

All of this was born out of insecurity, of course. And although natural, I realise now with time, age and knowledge that comparing ourselves to others is actually the biggest waste of our valuable time and energy.

Comparison is said to be the thief of joy. The moment we begin comparing ourselves to others, we become drawn into a negative interaction because someone always has to come out better or worse.

Dr Cotterill says: "There is absolutely no merit in comparison-related behaviours. The best thing we can do is be proud of and lift up other people, and focus on ourselves as an entirely separate entity. Our weight, appearance, wellbeing, health and eating habits are ours. We are where we are due to a range of factors and experiences individual to us. It doesn't help to compare ourselves to someone else's individual journey or experience. We can choose to focus on accepting and appreciating ourselves for who we are right now, and being compassionate and supportive to ourselves for where we are on our own journey of accepting ourselves, because this is what matters."

I recently read a quote from author Matt Haig, which really stuck with me: "Never try to be cool. Never worry what the cool people think. Head for the warm people. Life is warmth. You'll be cool when you're dead."

I love this piece of advice because, in this digital age especially, it's all too easy to worry incessantly about what other people think. The constant barrage of carefully curated posts online can easily leave us feeling inadequate and "uncool", perpetuating a never-ending cycle of comparison and feeling shit about ourselves.

CURATING YOUR SOCIAL MEDIA FEED

One of the biggest things that helped me in my self-acceptance journey was when I took the time to curate my social media feed a few years ago (as briefly mentioned in Chapter 1), unfollowing people that contributed to this sense of me feeling shitty about myself, and following a whole bunch more plus-size babes – both people who look like me, and people who don't.

The reason I mention social media in particular here is because, compared to other outlets, we consume it at a much higher rate. Apparently, millennials check their phone up to 150 times a day. Yikes.

But what we can often forget is that – unlike the generations before us, who were bombarded with diet culture on a daily basis from TV ads and in magazines – we actually have a certain amount of control online over whose messages we allow into our world and whose we leave out. I like to think of social media as my own little self-curated bubble, and it's up to me who lives in it.

I think we also forget that we have a very powerful tool at our disposal to avoid comparison and negative body image: the unfollow button. I recommend you use this liberally on:

- People you only follow because they're attractive
- People who only share their highlight reel
- Accounts that make you feel bad about yourself
- Brands that show little or no diversity
- Food accounts you follow for weight-loss motivation
- Fitness accounts that only focus on aesthetic instead of how fitness *feels*

I would also advise you to tread with caution when it comes to some of the people in the body-positive space online. I'm talking about people like the small, conventionally attractive women who, as mentioned in the previous chapter, sometimes distort their bodies to make it look like they have rolls when, in reality, they have none. Such people often don't have your best interests at heart.

The thing that it's important we remember about social media is that it's a platform, or "stage", which means that 90% of what we see on a person's feed is just a performance, rather than people's actual lives. As such, it's all the more ridiculous when we choose to compare ourselves to what we see on there, as what's the point in comparing our "inside" to someone else's "outside"?

So if you notice you are comparing yourself to others, instead:

- Take a breath.
- Notice your mind doing its comparing.
- Remind yourself gently that every person's situation is different to your own, so there's no benefit to comparing.
- Imagine completely letting go of all comparison thoughts. You might want to imagine them as words written on a balloon that is floating off into the sky. Every time the balloon floats back into sight, just let it drift off again.
- Bring your focus back to yourself and your day. What is important for you to focus on right here, right now?

HOW TO DEAL WITH NEGATIVE SELF-TALK

It's hard having to deal with other people's opinions (more on this in the next chapter), but sometimes our biggest critic is ourselves. The self-critical voice in our heads is often an accumulation of early parental/caregiver voices, the taunts of childhood bullies and/or the negative media narrative relating to weight and appearance.

This negative voice can tell you that your body is not OK, that you are a failure for eating that cake, that you are useless, have no willpower, are fat, unattractive ... the list goes on. So, if you experience this voice, please know you're not alone.

When negative self-talk starts creeping in, it can be useful to:

- Take a moment to really notice the voice and what it's saying.
- Remind yourself that you don't have to listen to it or give it any power. Challenge its validity, as it's not the truth. It's just the perspective of a mean, biased bully.
- Understand that being compassionate to yourself by not paying attention to the voice is not a sign of weakness. It's actually a way of helping you become stronger.
- Remember that when you're self-critical, you're attacking yourself and putting yourself in a state of heightened awareness and potential threat. And guess what? That's more likely to lead to you feeling down and anxious.
- Ask yourself how you would talk to a friend, family member or child who was going through the same kind of self-critical thoughts. You'd probably offer them support and kindness, right? So why not extend that same support to yourself?

Last but not least, you might want to try repeating these affirmations:

- I am enough.
- I am worthy.
- I am doing my best.
- I am learning new ways to look after myself and my body each day.
- I am learning to be kind to myself.
- I accept myself and my body completely.

A SELF-ACCEPTANCE SUMMARY

As we wrap up this chapter on the road to self-acceptance, let's remember the incredible power of being kind to ourselves. This journey is all about personal growth, finding fulfilment and experiencing genuine happiness.

Here's a little reminder of some the key practical steps that we've covered in this chapter that will help with this:

1. **Get comfortable with the mirror:** Stop picking yourself apart and start appreciating the person you see reflecting back at you. Let go of society's standards and acknowledge yourself as you are.
2. **Be comfortable taking up space:** Recognise your worth and own it. Stand tall, express your opinions and make your presence felt. You have every right to be seen and heard, just as you are.
3. **Don't compare yourself to others:** Instead, embrace your individuality, celebrate your unique strengths and achievements, and focus on your own happiness and growth.
4. **Carefully curate your social media feed:** Surround yourself with positive and inspiring content. Choose accounts and platforms that uplift and empower you. Unfollow accounts that don't make you feel good.

5. **Stop talking shit about yourself:** Challenge negative self-talk and replace it with words of kindness and affirmation.

I'm not going to lie to you and say that the road to self-acceptance is easy. Nor will I pretend that it happens overnight. In a society that profits from us having self-doubt, accepting and liking ourselves can almost feel like a rebellious act.

We've lost so many years of our lives to the grey haze that comes with being obsessed with our appearance. So let's not keep doing it.

We can do so much more than diet culture would ever want us to believe. So next time you start comparing yourself to others, or negative self-talk creeps in, remember that the body you've been taught to hate is truly your greatest friend.

SELF-EMPOWERMENT TASK

Take a little time out for yourself and try and remember a time, as a child, when you were particularly happy. You can even draw her on your notepad if you want, complete with a cape or a crown to show just how special she is.

Next time you talk shit about yourself, remember you're talking to her. How would she feel hearing all those mean things you're thinking? What impact would that have on her? What if you showed her unconditional acceptance, love and kindness instead?

9

Dealing with the weight of other people's opinions

How to respond and move forward with confidence

Now that we've looked at how we can be kinder to ourselves and avoid negative self-talk, it's time to look at how we deal with comments from outside sources. Because whether they're from strangers or people we know and love, they suck.

I don't know about you, but whenever a comment is made about my weight or general appearance, I feel almost paralysed by shock at first. It's like a punch to the gut. Then, shortly after that, comes the upset and anger. Sometimes it's as if there's heat rising inside of me. My cheeks turn pink, my stomach does a little flip-flop and my palms get all clammy. In less than two seconds of it happening, I'm busy praying for the ground to swallow me up, or planning my escape route.

I usually try and think of a witty comeback, but I just. can't. find. the. words. That's until later in the day or week, of course, when I replay the conversation over and over in my head, overanalyse every detail and act out different scenarios in which I do actually stick up for myself and say something really cutting or clever. "Why didn't I think of that sooner?!"

In the run-up to my wedding in 2017, a lot of people I cared about made inappropriate comments about my weight, and implied that I needed to "shred for the wed". One friend suggested I go on the Cambridge diet to "lose the weight fast". A woman at work told me: "If you don't lose it now, you never will." And even a very close family member said they'd pay for my wedding if I lost half of my body weight.

The truth is, no matter our size or shape, we've probably all experienced unwanted comments about our appearance at some point in our lives. Unfortunately, for reasons beyond me, some people feel it's their moral duty to pass judgement on our appearance and tell us if we've gained or lost weight.

I remember one Christmas day at home, my nan announced in front of the entire family how shocked she was at the amount of weight my stepsister had put on. For reference, my stepsister was only 15 and, not that it matters, but she'd put on a fair bit of weight due to going on the pill. She ran upstairs in floods of tears, as anyone would, and I remember asking my nan what she thought gave her the right to humiliate a vulnerable teenager in such a public way. She responded with: "I'm old, I can say what I like." Well, sorry, nan, but bollocks to that. Age does not give you a license to be a dick.

While my stepsister and I can laugh about it now, the truth is that these types of comments can leave a lasting mark on us and really affect our self-esteem.

Sometimes, I think criticisms from friends and relatives can hurt even more than ones from strangers, as it's particularly hard when the people who are meant to be in charge of *building* your self-confidence are the ones smashing it into a gazillion pieces. And it's even more tricky when derogatory comments are made under the guise of "I'm just worried about your health".

In spring 2023, singer, songwriter and actress Ariana Grande had to ask people to stop talking about her body and her health online, after "concerned" fans trolled her repeatedly about her weight loss. The general consensus was that she was "too skinny" and now an "unhealthy weight".

"There are many different ways to look healthy and beautiful," Grande said in the video she posted. "I know personally, for me, the body you've been comparing my current body to was the unhealthiest version of my body." She added that the physique fans were positioning as her "natural state" was actually a result of poor diet, antidepressants and generally being in a really low place in her life, before asking people to be gentler, and less comfortable talking about people's bodies.

She makes a good point. As a society we've gotten too comfortable commenting on other people's bodies, celebrity or not, and I think we need to become a bit more UNcomfortable doing so.

We need to realise that what other people look like is none of our damn business. Fat. Thin. Tall. Short. If it's not your body, it's not yours to comment on.

So, in this chapter, I want to give you some practical guidance on how to cope and what to say when difficult situations do crop up, so that you feel better equipped to deal with inappropriate comments and put boundaries in place.

HOW TO DEAL WITH NEGATIVE COMMENTS FROM OTHERS

There's no two ways about it. Negative comments from others about our weight, appearance or eating habits are unkind, and they hurt. They bring sadness, anxiety, embarrassment, guilt, anger, fear and shame.

So, it's important that we understand that our bodies, our appearance and our eating habits really are no one else's business. Even family or loved ones who "care'" about us simply have no right to comment on such matters unsolicited, as even when their comments are well-meaning, they tend to just leave us feeling bad about ourselves. As such, unsolicited advice or comments are simply never welcome or appropriate.

If you do experience unkind or negative comments coming your way, please know that:

- These comments are not OK. No one has a right to make comments about your appearance or make you feel bad about yourself. Period.
- It's not a "you" problem, it's a "them" problem. Often, people say things out of insecurity – because they're feeling bad about themselves and projecting. In your mind, try and place the responsibility back on them.
- Words hurt. You are allowed to notice, name and acknowledge the hurt for yourself, remembering to place the narrative firmly where it belongs (with the other person), e.g. "I feel very hurt and sad by that comment. That person has no place to comment on me/my body."
- You have a right to explain to the person who said the comments how they made you feel: "I found that comment really hurtful, so would ask you to not comment on my weight/appearance/eating from here on in, as I find it really triggering."

- Even if the person is a close family member or friend who claims to be saying something out of "concern" or "care", it is still OK to know that, unless you have asked for their opinion, you do not have to welcome or accept it.

One thing I like to do, if and when the subject of my weight is brought up, is firstly consider whether I feel it's coming from a place of kindness or cruelty. Of course, I know that, whatever the answer to that question is, no one has a right to comment on my body in the first place. But for me, I think it makes a huge difference if I ascertain the other person's intention first.

If someone is very obviously out to cause me shame or embarrassment with their comments, I will put a stop to it immediately by confronting them or walking away.

If someone comes to me with apparent "concerns" about my health, I try and determine how genuine their concern is and whether I feel there is truth in it. If someone is *genuinely* concerned about my health, they might say something like "I know this is a really sensitive subject, but I've noticed you've been hiding food recently/eating more than normal/avoiding dinner times. Is everything OK?" And this would, of course, be very different from someone saying something like "Should you really be eating that?", "I think you've had enough mashed potato for one day, don't you?", or "You really shouldn't wear that. It does nothing for you."

I know it's a cliché, but it's really important to be kind to yourself and use your self-compassion to tell yourself things like: "That comment makes me feel bad about myself, but I know I'm learning to accept myself and take care of myself. I cannot control the unkind comments of others, but I can choose to let them go and not let them take up my time and headspace. Their comments say more about them than about me." If the negative and/or cruel words keep playing on your mind, clinical psychologist Dr Emma Cotterill explains: "You can learn to notice these negative/cruel/critical thoughts and recognise when they are being unkind rather than compassionate. Once you have identified this, you can learn to choose to let these go rather than hold on to them. One way to do this is to imagine letting them drift away in the breeze – let them drift away, so that you are no longer burdened by their weight. They might float back, but you can then practise letting them float away again."

TIPS FOR WHEN SMALL TALK GETS DIET-Y

1. Change the subject as soon as you can. "Hey, have you seen that new show on Netflix?"

If it continues …

2. Tell them you're working on your relationship with food and would appreciate it if they didn't talk about diets, food or anything weight-related.

If it *still* continues …

3. Share some information about diet culture and how harmful it is. "Our food choices don't make us either good or bad, you know. Wouldn't it be awful if they did?"

If they're not getting the message …

4. Get more direct and tell them the conversation is making you uncomfortable.

If they're *still* not getting the message …

5. Remove yourself from the situation and send a clear message that you don't want to be part of this conversation.

SELF-EMPOWERMENT TASK

Take any hurtful words that others say to you and imagine them being sung to the tune of "Happy Birthday", spoken by Mickey Mouse, or rapped. Imagine them written in massive neon letters or bouncing around on a bouncing ball. The idea here is to make them seem as silly, ridiculous and meaningless as possible – until they no longer hurt.

Alternatively, or additionally, imagine yourself wearing steel armour, with any negative comments literally bouncing off you like arrows. Remember – they are just words, so it's up to you what you do with them.

WHAT TO SAY WHEN SOMEONE COMMENTS ON YOUR WEIGHT

Let's now have a look at some of the most common examples of weight-related comments that bigger-bodied people hear – and ways to respond to them.

It's important to acknowledge here that you may not feel confident enough to speak up and advocate for yourself all the time. And that's OK. You're not always going to think of the perfect comeback on the spot, and you're not weak if you aren't yet ready to retaliate at all. But my hope is that these examples might make you feel just that little bit pluckier the next time your weight comes up as a topic of conversation. You might want to amend a few to make them feel more "yours", memorise a few to keep in your back pocket, or come up with some alternatives of your own that you feel would work better for you.

"You'd be so pretty if you lost weight."
"That's really inappropriate and I don't appreciate you commenting on my weight or physical appearance. Please do not do that again."

"You look different. Have you gained weight?"
"That comment doesn't make me feel good at all. I have a history of struggling with food, so please don't ever comment on my weight or physical appearance."

"I've just joined a diet club and lost 10 pounds. You should try it."
"I'm happy that you're happy, but I'm actually working on making peace with my body and food, so I'd rather you didn't bring things like that up."

"Do you really need to eat that?"
"Absolutely! And I don't appreciate you commenting on my eating habits."

"You can't still be hungry."
"I think I know when I'm hungry and when to listen to my body's hunger signals, thanks."

"Is there something more flattering you could wear?"
"You saying things like that makes me feel really bad about myself when I think I look really good in this outfit. If you don't like it, don't wear it."

"I'm just worried about your health."
"You commenting on my weight doesn't motivate me or help me to be healthy. It actually does the opposite, so please don't do it."

WHAT TO SAY TO OTHER WEIGHT-RELATED THINGS THAT PEOPLE SAY

"I feel so fat today."

"Fat is not a feeling. Do you mean you feel bloated? Or is there something deeper going on?"

"I really need to go on a diet."

"I'm probably the wrong person to talk to about this. You know I love you no matter what you eat or what size you are."

"I deserve this treat. I've been really good today."

"You know our food choices don't make us good or bad, right? So why not just be kind to yourself? That's what I'm trying to do."

"Have you noticed how much weight [insert name here] has put on?"

"You seem to spend a lot of time talking about other people's body weight/shape/size. Why is that? And do you think it's helpful to anyone?"

DEALING WITH THE REACTIONS OF OTHERS AFTER WEIGHT GAIN

As already discussed, weight gain can happen for a whole range of different reasons, as well as for no apparent reason at all some times. But the stigma and shame – and even comments and looks from people in your life – that come with it is often universal.

As someone who has *always* existed in a bigger body, I wanted to enlist the help of someone who experienced weight gain in *later* life to share what it's like and offer advice on how to deal with comments about it.

This is my best friend and podcast co-host Lauren's story:

For me, although I'd always been the biggest of my friends, I was still only a UK size 12 [US size 8] until I was 26. When I celebrated my 30th birthday, I was wearing a UK size 20 [US size 16] because, after something traumatic happened when I was 27, I overate and binged as a way to cope with it. I didn't realise this until years later, but food became something I could control at a time when my world was falling apart.

Similarly to most people whose bodies change in this way, I felt all the stigma and pressure the world told me I should be feeling for having "let myself go". So I spent years leaning into that: hiding away at home, not posing for photos, covering my body in jeans and cardigans in the summer, wearing black, baggy clothes to hide my growing body, and refusing to buy the clothes I really liked because being fat was only temporary, right? I was starting that new diet on Monday, so I'd be skinny again soon.

The backdrop of all these feelings was the memory of how the world treated me when I was slimmer. The bigger I got, the more I realised that this world wasn't made for me anymore. And that was heartbreaking.

For example, as a single, straight woman, I would see the way men would look through me, not at me, on nights out with my friends. Things like this killed my confidence even more. I would stand awkwardly in Zara as my friends picked up beautiful outfits that, not long before, I would have fitted into with ease. Now it was clear I wasn't welcome at that shop, and a number of shops, anymore. I would try to smile as compliments changed from "Wow, you look great in that dress" to "Wow, you have such a pretty face" or "Doesn't your hair look lovely?". I was petrified of bumping into an ex or someone from school and seeing the inevitable look in their eyes.

Your world suddenly becomes smaller and harder, and so much is different. But although your body has changed, you haven't. You're still the same person you were before, you're just wearing bigger clothes now.

And that's when I realised that, although the size of my knickers had changed, I hadn't. I was still as kind and clumsy, smart and loud, and considerate and crass as I'd always been. My worth hadn't changed, even though my dress size had, and that realisation changed everything for me.

I refused to let myself shrink into a smaller life that I didn't want just because of what others thought of my body. I hadn't "let myself go", I'd had an ordinary response to an extraordinary thing. Yes, my body looks different to how it did when I was 22. And how normal is that!

Slowly, I started to transform my wardrobe into a sea of colourful dresses, mirroring what I'd always enjoyed wearing before. I started saying "yes" to more, I chose to be in photos, I made memories, I dated, I travelled, I took chances and I stopped treating myself as if I were temporary.

Think of the next five years of your life; think of all the memories and fun and experiences you might be missing out on if you hide yourself away. Don't wait until you "lose the weight". Start living again now.

One of the best pieces of advice I've ever been given on how to accept my body was about learning to see it as desirable, sexy and confident at the size it is now. Because learning to accept and appreciate your current body will help you realise just how worthy and wonderful you are. Give it a try – walk around your house naked, look in the mirror, take photos, treat yourself to *lingerie. It doesn't have to be anything too much, whatever you're comfortable with and confident in.*

Although we may miss the way the world treated us when we were in smaller bodies, please don't let that stop you living a full and happy life. Because you're still the same person, just in bigger pants.

HOW SHOULD YOU COMMENT ON SOMEONE ELSE'S WEIGHT?

The correct time to comment on someone's weight is never.

Why? Because, on the whole, it tells the person that their size or appearance is one of the most important aspects about them and, depending on what you say, it potentially also tells them that they hold more value in a smaller body. However, not complimenting someone when they have lost weight is something that even I still find difficult, as it's so ingrained in us to *celebrate* being a smaller size!

I recently bumped into the mum of a friend of mine. I knew that she'd lost a lot of weight due to an underlying health condition, and yet I had to stop myself from saying "You look great, you've lost so much weight". It takes years to unlearn the things diet culture has ingrained in us. But the thing is that, when we compliment weight loss, we could unknowingly be complimenting an eating disorder, a medical issue or a trauma such as a divorce or a loss.

I recently carried out a poll online asking women if they'd been complimented for their weight loss when they were actually dealing with something traumatic, and 66% of them said yes. Here are some of the thousands of responses:

- "I was struggling with post-natal depression after the birth of my daughter."
- "I could barely eat due to the stress of law school exams; I was petrified of gaining it back for fear of what people would say."
- "I was grieving a horrible loss."
- "I was depressed and not eating."
- "I lost 5 stone (70 lb/32 kg) and found out I had Crohn's disease; everyone said how healthy I looked."
- "I got divorced and stopped eating; apparently divorce 'suited me'."
- "I had a miscarriage and couldn't eat; first day back in the office after three weeks, and got told how good I looked."
- "I was suicidal."

I don't think it's necessarily our fault for being so interested in body size. We've been conditioned all our lives by diet culture and the media to derive our worth from our looks, and this is a problem that's been passed down from one generation to the next.

Dr Cotterill says: "When we comment or compliment someone's weight loss, we are emphasising appearance and reinforcing the social narratives that weight loss is important and of significant value (at the detriment to other things such as our physical and mental health)." And, while compliments may provide a momentary boost in mood, they are actually unhelpful in the long run because they can lead to us associating feeling good with being told we have lost weight/are slim, which might make us focus on achieving these compliments at the detriment of our health. They can also make us feel bad if we gain weight and *don't* get compliments any more.

Complimenting someone on their shrinking frame really is problematic for many reasons. For example, it can reinforce unhealthy behaviours, and can actually intensify food restriction, excessive exercise or other such self-punishing behaviour. As Dr Cotterill says, "There are so many other ways that we can compliment someone or so many other qualities that we can recognise as valuable and important about a person – how good it is to see them, how they are taking care of themselves (self-care), their values (e.g. kindness, thoughtfulness) or achievements, resilience, or things to be proud of in life, work, family, etc."

What I tend to say now if friends have lost weight and comment on it from their side, is "And are you feeling well?" And if they say yes, I say: "Then I'm happy for you."

Shutting down weight-centred comments even in ways as kind and gentle as this delivers the message that you do not value a fixation on body size. Plus, it potentially also gets the other person thinking about why they *do* value body size to such a great extent. And that is what starts the cycle of change in wider society.

ESTABLISHING BOUNDARIES AROUND WEIGHT AND DIET TALK

Let's face it. There are times in our lives when we just know that weight comments are going to come flooding in. Family members can often feel the need to comment on our bodies (or other people's) and make comments about food choices.

In the past, a cruel comment or even a backhanded compliment about my body had a habit of lodging itself in my memory and resurfacing when I was feeling particularly crappy. Although both of these things can be difficult, there are things that we can do to prepare ourselves in advance. For example, you might consider sending a text in advance of an event, explaining your concerns and feelings around diet talk and weight-related comments, and how you would really appreciate it if the subjects of dieting or foods being good or bad were not brought up.

I recently heard from a listener of my podcast who wrote a letter to her dad and stepmum after noticing how fixated they were on what they were eating and the amount of calories they were consuming. They had recently found out that he had high cholesterol, so were trying to get that down by eating "clean" (i.e. no processed foods, no sugar, no carbs) and in a calorie deficit.

In her letter, she said she was really happy for her dad's new-found passion for food and exercise, but that she was trying to educate her children to not think about food as good or bad, and not fixate on what they were eating or their weight. She asked politely if they could be mindful of this when they visited next. Despite being really nervous about offending her dad, his response was extremely understanding, and he actually appreciated the heads-up because he hadn't realised how obsessive he and his wife had become about it. All in all, then, writing the letter in an understanding, respectful way – while also making her boundaries clear – meant for a happy outcome.

Of course, this is the ideal scenario, and it's important to note that some interactions, whether spoken or written, will be a lot messier than this. Nonetheless, it goes to show that a conversation really can be worth having, and it may not even end up being as scary as you think. It's still important we put boundaries in place, even if we fear that the response won't be positive.

If a letter feels too formal or too scary, you could try a more casual text instead, such as:

Hey! How are you? This might seem a bit out of the blue, but I just wanted to give you a heads-up that I'm doing a lot of work on my relationship with food at the moment, so please can we refrain from talking about diets, etc. when we meet? I'd really appreciate it. Thanks!

Remember, not everyone will be on board with your new freedoms – some people are (and perhaps always will be) caught up in the wrath of diet culture. You can't win everyone round, but you certainly can try.

Sharing a little education can go a long way, so sometimes, I gently point people in the direction of books I've read or podcasts I've listened to about diet culture and the negative impact it has. If people are open to it, great. If not, you tried.

SAYING GOODBYE TO THE NEED FOR APPROVAL

This is easier said than done, I know. But there comes a time when you have to own who you are and not be at the mercy of other people's opinions. For me, that means accepting that I will probably always be in a bigger body, and that that's OK – even if my nan or my mum or my great aunt Sally don't think it is.

You don't owe anyone thinness. And it is not your life's purpose to be "attractive" to others. And, while you can't control some of the responses you get from other people about your body, whether in real life or online, you *can* control how you feel and respond to them.

My advice for the next time someone comments on your body?

1. Remember that people's perceptions are subjective and, more often than not, inaccurate. They're not a true reflection of who you are. As mentioned earlier, they're also likely to be a projection of their own insecurities.
2. Rather than feeling devastated or diminished, try to see the bigger picture and have an objective understanding of the way you look and the person you are.
3. Don't be afraid to speak up in order to nip negative remarks in the bud when people overstep the mark. Every unwelcome comment can be a chance for you to share your definition of what is and isn't acceptable as commentary on *your* body. Society is on the turn; so many people should know by now that it's not OK to talk about people's bodies.
4. Try to move on. Think about what you love about yourself – and remember, the way you look is the least interesting thing about you. You know in your heart your many positive and interesting qualities – none of which have anything to do with how much you weigh.

Crucially, I want you to know, above all else, that nothing and no one is more important than your mental health, even if that means cutting people out of your life who continue to disrespect your wishes and boundaries.

SELF-EMPOWERMENT TASK

Take some time out for yourself and think about someone you admire for their confidence. It can be a celebrity, a fictional character or someone you know in real life.

Then, when you're next in a situation where you're struggling with judgement from other people, ask yourself: what would this "confidence role model" do?

Would *they* put up with people making shitty comments to them? Or would they stand up for themselves?

Try to gain strength and inspiration from what you feel they would do, and roll with it ...

10

Reframing your relationship with exercise

Bringing the joy back into movement

I have always associated exercise with one thing: punishment. For a long time, I believed that exercise was a way to simply "earn" food and burn calories. If I wasn't beetroot red and on the verge of a heart attack at the end of a gym session, I wasn't doing it "right", in my mind.

I remember going to my local gym as a teenager and slogging it out on the treadmill for what felt like hours – bored out of my brain and watching intently as the number of calories burned went up at a painfully slow rate. I also remember, during one particularly horrendous PE lesson at school, being made to run track. The only other chubby girl in my class and I were lagging behind at the back and thought it would be funny to chant the number to Childline at the top of our voices over and over again. To be fair, I still think that's pretty funny. But you get the gist. Me and exercise were not friends.

I really envied people, like my brother, who took naturally to sports. He was athletic, slim, good at everything – a natural athlete and team leader. Whereas everything I tried, I gave up on within a week.

The assumption was that I was lazy. And to be fair, I was. But it was more than that. Even at a young age, my body didn't feel "suitable" for gymnastics, ballet or even swimming – a sport that I loved and felt at home in. Part of the problem was also that I really disliked having to wear a swimming costume, a leotard or shorts. I felt like a fat freak and was worried about being bullied even more than I already was.

Every attempt at exercise was just another reminder for me of what my body *couldn't* do and how big it was, i.e. *too* big.

It was really only a few years ago (not long after I turned 30) that my relationship with exercise started to change when I fell back in love with swimming (more on this later in this chapter). I don't claim to have it all figured out now (give me a day on the sofa wrapped in a blanket like a burrito over a sweaty gym workout any day). But I do feel like I'm doing a good job of gradually healing my relationship with exercise, and I really want that for you, too.

EXERCISE AS THE ENEMY?

If you're reading this and have a complex relationship with exercise, the first thing I want you to know is that it's not your fault. I also want you to know that this is incredibly common, given that so many of us have had negative experiences with exercise in the past. You may, for example, have been punished at school by being made to do 100 burpees, or you may have been made to do certain sports activities as a way to "toughen you up".

Personally, I think a lot of my issues around exercise come from it having been forced on me by my parents as a way solely to lose weight, rather than it ever feeling like it could have anything to do with enjoyment or fun. First, I was encouraged to play football (which I *hated*). I was so bad at it that I used to be put in goal, where I used to sing show tunes to pass the time! Then I was told that my body type was "perfect for shotput" (spoiler alert: I hated that too). I even remember being made to do obstacle courses around the garden in an attempt to get me moving more. But every attempt to make me more active failed. In fact, if anything, it just made me hate – and resent – exercise even more.

A 2023 study published in the journal *Appetite* found that negative experiences with exercise in childhood can not only lead to the creation of a negative association with movement in adulthood, but also disordered eating and body-image issues, too.

SELF-EMPOWERMENT TASK

Take a little time out for yourself and think back on your experience with exercise as a child. Did you enjoy it, or find it challenging? Did it revolve around play or organised sports? Did you have any role models who motivated you to engage in physical activity? If so, how did they influence your approach to exercise?

Looking back, how do you think your experiences with exercise as a child have shaped your attitudes and habits towards physical activity today?

Feel free to write down anything that feels particularly pertinent to you, such as attitudes that you might like to now let go of, in order to feel more liberated and/or empowered in your own body.

WHAT WE'RE TOLD FITNESS LOOKS LIKE

A huge factor that influences our thoughts and feelings about exercise is that most of us have been led to believe that fitness means a certain aesthetic. For years we've been told that how fit we are will directly correlate to what size we are and what we look like – with little margin for error. But that's simply not true. I want to make it really clear that you can't tell how fit someone is just from their appearance.

From fitness magazines to "What I eat in a day" videos on TikTok, we're bombarded with images of "perfect", "fit" bodies, and messages that tell us we're not good enough unless we look a certain way. This often creates a sense of inadequacy, which either makes us feel like we need to punish ourselves with exercise in order to measure up, or give up entirely.

We spoke a lot about the importance of representation in Chapter 4, but I want to reiterate here that I think the fitness industry is missing the mark when it comes to representing different body types. So many of us don't feel seen or included in the notion of fitness because the impression we get is that the fitness industry is an elitist club for folk that are able-bodied, skinny and wealthy. And let's be honest, it is a luxury of both time and money to be able to work out in a gym.

What's more, a lot of people (myself included) think that if they don't look like the people on the cover of a fitness magazine, or the fitness influencer they follow online, exercise isn't for them. And that can equate to being nervous about going to the gym because you feel like you have to be a certain size to even be worthy of going there.

For a while, I used to really love going to Zumba classes, but I've gone off it ever since one particular instructor kept making derogatory remarks about my stomach and telling me to "keep up".

A 2018 study conducted by researchers at Northwestern University in the US delved into the influence of fitness instructors' comments on women's body satisfaction. The study involved two groups of participants who took part in a 16-minute conditioning class. Both groups performed the same workout in the same environment, accompanied by identical music. However, the key difference was the instructor's choice of words for each group.

For one group, the instructor used motivational language that focused on the benefits of the exercises, such as building leg strength and enhancing performance in activities like running and jumping. The participants in this group reported feeling more positive about their bodies after the class, expressing a sense of accomplishment and strength.

In contrast, the other group received appearance-focused motivational comments from the instructor, centred around body shape and fat reduction. This group didn't experience the same positive emotions after their workout. In fact, when asked to describe their feelings at the end of the class, one said she felt "ashamed" and another even said she was "disgusted with [her]self".

The study shows that if we approach exercise as a means of "fixing" ourselves, which is generally linked to feelings of shame, guilt or maybe even punishment, then it can actually *harm* our mental health. But it doesn't need to be this way.

WHAT FITNESS CAN *ACTUALLY* LOOK (AND FEEL) LIKE

It's time to let go of fitness stereotypes and be more creative and open-minded when it comes to moving our bodies. We don't *have* to look a certain way, have an expensive gym membership or wear trendy workout shoes as a status symbol in order to enjoy movement in our life and get fitter.

Fitness is not an aesthetic. And guess what? It can actually be fun.

We often have the idea that a good workout is one that leaves us sweating profusely and half dead on the floor, or that we need to exercise for a minimum amount of time for it to be effective. But the truth is that a good workout is one that you enjoy and sustain. One that makes you feel empowered and brings you joy.

Getting to know your own motivating factors when it comes to exercise is so important, as it's this that allows us to firmly frame fitness as something that enhances our lives, rather than being about our appearance. So, think for a moment: what about exercise *do* you, or *could* you, enjoy? The fact that it gives you more energy to play with your kids? That it gives you a sweet dopamine hit? That it gets you out in the fresh air?

There can be so many amazing benefits to exercise and movement, including increased strength, better quality of sleep and even lower stress levels. Why shouldn't those of us in bigger bodies benefit from all of these things?

BARRIERS TO FITNESS

One big gripe I have with the fitness industry is how hard it is to find decent plus-size activewear, with most brands stopping at a UK size 18 (US size 14).

Nike (who, by the way, do great plus-size gym gear) hit the headlines in 2019 over their introduction of plus-size mannequins at their flagship store in London. While many saw this as a positive step towards inclusivity, a lot of people were outraged and accused Nike of promoting obesity (major eye roll).

The irony here is that the critics of Nike said they should focus on encouraging people to lose weight and get fit, rather than promoting a "fat-acceptance" agenda. But surely, providing clothing for bigger people does just that?

If the fatphobic twats of the world are so hell-bent on fat people exercising and getting fitter, what do they suggest we work out in? Our birthday suit?!

Maybe brands just don't want bigger people wearing their clothes, I don't know. But I do know that a lack of suitable, and nice, fitness clothes can be a barrier to us feeling the part and showing up, and I'm sure we can all agree that that isn't good.

RECLAIMING EXERCISE FROM HUSTLE CULTURE

In addition to the lack of inclusivity and access to clothing, I often wonder if some of our issues around exercise are because of the way in which Western society places such a high value on productivity and achievement – often to the detriment of our health and wellbeing.

This focus on "hustle culture" teaches us to work ever harder and longer, even if it's at the expense of sleep, leisure time and physical activity.

And the constant pressure to "perform" can leave us feeling guilty or selfish if we take a lot of time out to exercise.

Tally Rye, inclusive personal trainer and author of the book *Train Happy*, says on this topic, "Whether it's diet culture or hustle culture, it's important to remember that our attitudes towards exercise are not our fault. We've been conditioned by years of cultural messaging that has emphasised the importance of appearance and achievement over health and wellbeing. We've been told that exercise is something we should do to punish ourselves for our perceived shortcomings, rather than something we should do to take care of our bodies and minds."

When you stop and think about it, a lot of what we associate with exercise is often tied in some way to numbers, whether calories burned, time spent or steps taken. So much so that we often end up quantifying our workouts by how much we "got" out of them rather than how they make us feel, which should surely be pretty important!

HEALING YOUR RELATIONSHIP WITH EXERCISE

So, what can we do to change this negative mindset towards exercise?

First, we need to start reframing our thoughts about it – so that, rather than thinking of exercise as any kind of punishment or necessary achievement, we begin to think of it as a way to nourish and care for our bodies. And maybe even as a celebration of what your body *can* do, and an opportunity to feel and grow stronger and fitter.

Second, we need to focus less on appearance-based goals and more on how exercise makes us *feel* – whether that's being more energised, more relaxed or generally happier.

WHAT KIND OF MOVER ARE YOU?

The chart below, created by inclusive personal trainer Tally Rye, shows three main different types of "movers": All or Nothing, Rigid, and Intuitive. Have a read through each column and see which one most resonates with you, to get a quick overview of your current relationship with exercise. Then, have a think about whether you are happy with this or would like to make some changes …

All or Nothing	Rigid	Intuitive
Exercise linked with dieting/"health kicks" but never lasts once the diet stops	Pushes through pain, injury and illness to complete scheduled exercise	Chooses workouts that feel good and are enjoyable
Exercise associated with pain, discomfort and punishment, so generally avoided	Feels guilt and fear for unplanned rest days	Focuses on supporting physical and mental wellbeing, not on weight/aesthetics
Works out for upcoming events/holidays, etc., but stops afterwards	MUST track all workouts/steps and complete activity goals on fitness watch	Recognises that energy levels vary and moves body in accordance with that
Relies on extrinsic motivation because you "should"	Selects workouts based on calorie burn	Allows for flexibility and rest even when working towards fitness goals
	Schedule/social life revolves around workouts	Fit is a feeling and not a body type

Box text copyright Tally Rye (@tallyrye)

INTRODUCING INTUITIVE MOVEMENT

While it may sometimes feel like the odds are stacked against us, the good news is that having a better relationship with exercise *is* possible.

In recent years, there has been a real shift away from gruelling gym sessions, towards something known as "intuitive movement". If you haven't heard of it before, intuitive movement offers a more gentle and flexible approach to exercise than traditional approaches, which tend to focus on rigid routines and strict rules.

Intuitive movement encourages us to find joy in movement, listen to our bodies and honour their unique needs at any given time. This means that if you fancy doing a two-hour run one day, you can. But if all you're up to is a 10-minute walk around the park another day, then that's fine too. All movement is valid, and all movement is good.

Intuitive movement is about developing a deep connection with the body and learning to trust its signals and cues. It involves tuning into our physical sensations, emotions and energy levels, and allowing *these* to guide our movement choices. The idea is that by really listening to our bodies and responding with compassion, we can create a more sustainable and fulfilling exercise routine that supports our overall health and wellbeing.

Sounds good, right?

In the words of Rye, "Intuitive movement can be pretty life-changing when it comes to your relationship with moving your body. It means you don't have to dread working out and you don't have to make fitness your whole identity through regimented exercise, either. There is a place where you can listen and work *with* your body from a place of self-care and respect."

Intuitive movement is a framework that has been designed to help you rebuild your relationship with exercise so that, instead of being about weight, aesthetics and trying to control your body, it's about supporting your health (both physical and mental) and, most importantly, having fun! This way, you're more likely to be able to develop a relationship with exercise that's both consistent and sustainable in the long term. Needless to say, I'm a fan!

Rye explains that "so many people get stuck in a very 'all-or-nothing' cycle with exercise and they swing between completely overdoing it – thinking that exercise must always be really intense – and then, naturally, they burn out because that's not sustainable."

Instead, Rye works with her clients to uncover their own "effort scale" when it comes to exercise, which involves considering what different levels of physical effort feel like on a scale of 0 to 10 to them. Her clients often start off believing that their effort level must be above a 7/10 for anything they're doing to be counted as "proper exercise", and that they have to be sore, exhausted and sweaty after a "good workout"!

But Rye urges them to stop judging their exercise in this way and instead to find a level of physical activity that feels sustainable and enjoyable for *them* at any given time. This might mean starting with low-impact activities, such as walking or yoga, or finding a form of exercise that feels fun and engaging, such as dancing or swimming. And the effort level can – and should – constantly vary: "Through intuitive movement, the goal is for people to find physical activity that spans across all levels of the effort scale."

For those of us with a tendency towards an all-or-nothing approach when it comes to exercise, or who have had a tumultuous or extreme relationship with exercise in the past, Rye urges us to remember that intense exercise is not the only way to benefit from physical activity. She warns: "Jumping back in at a high level like 7, 8, 9 or 10 may not be the best approach. Instead, try to find a level of activity that falls within the 0 to 6 range and gradually build confidence and consistency from there."

FINDING MOVEMENT YOU ENJOY

Now that we know that moving our body intuitively, without a need for extremes, is a healthy way to go, it's time to consider HOW we want to introduce more movement into our lives. So let's start by having a little look back at exercise trends over the last few decades …

Back in the '80s, Jane Fonda's aerobics videos led the way in a high-energy, high-impact exercise trend that was all about burning calories and sculpting a "perfect" body. The '90s brought further high-energy trends such as spinning, Tae Bo and step aerobics. And the early 2000s then ushered in the era of practices such as yoga and Pilates. More recently, there's been a surge in interest in high-intensity interval training (HIIT), which involves short bursts of intense exercise followed by periods of rest.

While all of these are great in their own way, the problem with any trend is that they're all about what's new and "most effective", rather than about what you actually *enjoy*. So, here's an important question for you: do you know what you actually like? Or have you always just been caught up in trying whatever trends the fitness industry has pushed your way?

As I briefly mentioned earlier, swimming has always been a favourite form of exercise for me. (Think of me as a fat, white version of Disney's Moana.) I have some amazing memories of holidays abroad, where my dad would spin me around in the water and do handstands with me. He adored the water, and so did I, as a child. Swimming didn't even feel like exercise when I was young. So, it makes me incredibly sad to think that I gave it up in my teenage years because I was too self-conscious of being in a swimming costume in public.

Fortunately, however, I rediscovered my love for it when, a few years ago, my husband Matt and I booked an impromptu trip to the Lake District and experienced open-water swimming for the first time. We went for a night-time swim in the pouring rain – in muddy water that completely battered us because of the gale-force winds. But I absolutely loved it. So much so that I decided to book an induction at a lake near where I lived and started doing it regularly. It was a struggle to find a wetsuit that fitted, and I have to admit that concerns about looking like a Teletubby crept in. But, thankfully, my love for swimming and my desire to be in the water were bigger than my fears about how I would look while doing it.

I can honestly say that it's one of the best things I've ever done for myself. The feeling I have when I'm in the water is like no other. I feel weightless, happy and free. I'm just so grateful I gave swimming another chance, and that I've finally found a form of exercise that I can not only do, but that I enjoy and makes me feel great!

I think for a long time we've been conditioned to think that going to the gym and sweating it out on the treadmill is the only real way to work out. But it truly is all about finding what you like – and then sticking to it. As Rye says: "People often follow the latest on-trend workout or what their personal trainer at the gym recommends. Enjoyment never really comes into the equation. But I think people are now burnt out from that."

When Rye begins coaching a new client, she asks them to list every single way they can think of to move their body. This includes everything from ballet, hula-hooping and dancing around the kitchen to open-water swimming, rock climbing and skiing. The full kaleidoscope of movement!

She then encourages them to really figure out what they enjoy through a trial-and-error process and get playful …

REMEMBERING THE REAL BENEFITS OF EXERCISE

Here's a question for you: if exercise had ZERO impact on your weight or appearance, would you still do it? I think we often forget that the real benefits of exercise have nothing to do with being smaller or having a perky bum. So, it's important that we shift our mindset towards remembering that exercise benefits our overall health – mental as well as physical.

Lizzo spoke about this in a 2023 TikTok video and it really resonated with me. She said how "weight loss comes with the territory" of working out, but wasn't, for her, an attempt to "escape fatness": "I think a lot of people see a fat person that way and immediately just assume everything they are doing is trying to be thin. I'm not trying to be thin. I don't ever want to be thin."

"The goal is always *here*," she said, pointing to her head, before explaining that exercise had helped shift her mind – not her body. And she's absolutely right. Have you ever, for example, stepped on the scales after a week of healthy eating and exercise, only to see that the number hasn't budged? Yet you still feel better overall, as you have more energy or maybe your clothes are fitting better?

As I hope you've realised as you've read this book, weight is just a number – not an accurate measure of health. What's more, constantly weighing ourselves can, and often does, lead to an unhealthy preoccupation with weight and size. It certainly led *me* to develop disordered habits over the years. I remember being at university and feeling so desperate to lose weight that I was exercising constantly and eating nothing but eggs and drinking orange juice. I weighed myself at least twice a day, and revelled in seeing the number go down drastically. Until, all of a sudden, it didn't. At which point, I started to obsess over every little fluctuation and became even more of a slave to the scales. The combination of continual, intense exercise and extreme food restriction wasn't sustainable for me, of course, so I binged when I felt like a failure and put on all the weight I lost.

I wish I could go back and tell my younger self that there are so many better ways to track your progress and focus on your overall health than weighing yourself! Dr Joshua Wolrich suggests using methods such as monitoring energy levels, strength gains and improvements in mood. He says: "Regular movement is amazing for your health, but many people only start doing it because they've been told it will help them lose weight. When this doesn't happen, activity levels often drop. Making health all about weight is not only nonsense, but it can actually lead to people disregarding behaviours that are really good for them." So, next time you get the urge to weigh yourself, why not try measuring your progress by how you *feel* instead? Are you feeling stronger? More energetic? Happier? These are all signs that your body is responding positively.

FINDING YOUR INTUITIVE MOVEMENT SWEET SPOT

The radical swing from crash dieting and exercising compulsively to a "fuck it, I'll eat what I want" mentality is something I've done for pretty much my entire life. Maybe you have too? I was really interested to talk to personal trainer Tally Rye about this. She explained to me that there's a process we have to go through to get to the sweet spot with intuitive movement, which is what the diagram below, courtesy of her, sets out.

INTUITIVE MOVEMENT PENDULUM

START HERE

DIET MENTALITY PHASE
- Restriction
- Guilt & shame
- All-or-nothing approach
- Rigid mindset
- 'Should' work out
- Only weight/aesthetic-based goals

FINAL DESTINATION

INTUITIVE MOVEMENT SWEET SPOT
- Movement is self-care
- Rest without guilt
- Fitness is a feeling not a look
- Joyful movement
- Listen to the body
- Performance-based fitness goals
- Flexible structure/routine

STOP OFF HERE

F* IT PHASE**
- Little/no movement
- Reject diet mentality
- Rebel against old rules
- No structure
- Rest to recover

Copyright Tally Rye (@tallyrye) – from her book *The Train Happy Journal* (Pavilion, 2021)

As we can see from the diagram opposite, when we're in the pendulum swing of the "diet mentality", our approach to movement is all about restriction, guilt and shame, with an all-or-nothing approach that's very rigid.

Then, when you start to learn about diet culture and begin to unlearn its harmful messages, you're likely to swing to the "fuck-it" phase, which tends to involve little to no movement and a rejection of all your old "diet mentality" rules and restrictions (like only eating certain foods or exercising in a certain way). This often leads to a period of rebellion, where you indulge in all the things you were not previously "allowed" to eat or do.

Once you've shed one layer of diet culture, you may well find yourself swinging back to the "diet mentality" zone again, only to discover another layer of damaging beliefs and biases that you're still holding on to and need to let go of. It's possible that you might swing back and forward, from left to right for a while.

But eventually, you'll settle into a more balanced approach, in the middle – called the "intuitive movement sweet spot" – where you can enjoy movement and exercise as a form of self-care, without feeling like you're stuck in a rigid routine.

Note that resting and recovery are crucial parts of this process, especially if you have a history of disordered eating or excessive exercise habits. The length of breaks that you take between exercise sessions will depend on your individual circumstances and needs, but it's important to listen to your body and give yourself the time and space that you feel you need to heal and recover.

"The 'fuck-it' phase is an important part of the process and shouldn't be skipped or bypassed," says Rye. "It's OK to take longer in this phase, especially if this has been a big part of your life for a long time. Rome wasn't built in a day, and it wasn't dismantled in a day either. It's important to give yourself grace and compassion and acknowledge that you're figuring things out."

After you're revelled in the "fuck-it" phase for as long as you need, you might suddenly think it could be nice to move a bit, go for a walk, feel stronger … This is when you are likely to start to swing – slowly and mindfully – to the intuitive movement sweet spot in the middle, which is what we're aiming for.

But what does it look/feel like when we've found it?

- It's about understanding that movement is a form of self-care.
- We're able to rest without feeling guilty.
- We've realised that fitness is more about feeling than appearance.
- We've found joyful movement and know how to listen to our bodies.
- We may have performance-based fitness goals, but they're not based on aesthetics.
- We avoid setting strict schedules like "work out five days a week", which can cause us to spiral out of control when we miss a day. Instead, we aim for a nice equilibrium where missing a day is fine.

THE PENDULUM KEEPS MOVING

Rye's pendulum analogy, and the fact that pendulums keep moving – allows us to recognise that finding our intuitive movement sweet spot is an ongoing process. This means that it's very likely that you'll swing into "diet mentality" again and into the "fuck-it" phase again – and that doesn't mean you're a failure! Remember: you're undoing years of disordered thinking around exercise here, so you need to be kind to yourself as you try new things! But as the pendulum keeps moving, what you're likely to find is that the swing starts to have smaller and smaller movements until it finds its final "intuitive sweet spot" resting place.

While I may not be quite at the sweet spot yet, I've been trying really hard to improve my relationship with exercise over the years, and I feel like I'm now in a much better place than before. It genuinely wasn't until I realised that I didn't have to see exercise as a punishment that I started to shift the focus away from weight loss to the other benefits it can bring: building strength, increasing flexibility, reducing stress and improving my mental health, among other things.

As well as swimming, I now walk my dog Buddy for an hour every day and, while it's annoying on the days that it's cold and wet, there is an odd satisfaction I feel once I'm home.

I think it's likely I will always have a complex relationship with exercise. Being bigger means things are physically more challenging, too. But now that I know it's not all about weight, or punishment, or earning food, I know that there's nothing to be scared of.

I hope this chapter has helped you to learn about why you might feel the way you do about exercise, and that it encourages you to find joy in movement again and work towards your very own intuitive sweet spot.

Remember that fitness and health are not one-size-fits-all. Our bodies are unique, and what works for one person may not work for you. So focus on what feels good for you and your body, and take it one day at a time.

SELF-EMPOWERMENT TASK

Take a little time out for yourself and write down all the different forms of movement and exercise that you enjoy, or used to enjoy as a child. Then have a think about which of these you might *like* to incorporate, and be *able* to incorporate, into your regular routine.

Don't be afraid to think out of the box. If you hate the gym but love boxing, buy a punching bag and put it in your garden. If you hate running on the treadmill, why not try a walk or a hike instead? Alternatively, there might a new form of exercise that you've always wanted to try; if so, go for it. There are no rights or wrongs here. It's about finding what works best for you ...

11

Healing your relationship with food
A life without obsession and dieting?

I was on a spa break with a friend a couple of years ago when I overheard a woman talk about how she desperately wanted to have pasta for dinner (her favourite), but was too worried about the calories. She said she didn't want to leave her holiday heavier than when she came. In all honesty, it made me sad. Sad that, in her late 60s, this lovely woman felt she couldn't enjoy a bowl of pasta while on holiday because she was too worried about gaining weight. I don't know this woman's story and there was no judgement from me. It just got me thinking about how many of us have grappled with guilt when it comes to our food choices.

It made me think about the time, not that long ago, that actor Zac Efron nearly broke down in tears eating a big bowl of pasta during a Netflix documentary. "I'm so happy I'm eating carbs again," he said. "I went years without eating carbs. When I shot *Baywatch*, I didn't have a carb for six months. I almost lost my mind. You … you need this."

So, to the woman in the restaurant, to Zac and to you, I want to say this:

Food is not the enemy. Your body is not a battleground.
You deserve to feel nourished, in both body and soul.

In this chapter, we're therefore going to look at how to have a healthier relationship with food WITHOUT the need for dieting, and WITHOUT the nagging voice of diet culture telling you you're "good", "bad" or a complete waste of space.

A COMPLEX RELATIONSHIP

The truth is, our relationship with food is complex. The vast majority of women I spoke to during the writing of this book said they would class their relationship with it as "complicated" (88% in fact).

For many of us, food represents not just nourishment, but also comfort and pleasure. (My stepmum always used to say that some food is good for our health, while some food is good for our soul.) But, for lots of us, food can also be a source of anxiety, guilt and shame.

A 2005 study in the *Journal of Health and Social Behavior* found that 79% of fat people reported using food as a coping mechanism. Research has shown that our relationship with food is shaped by a variety of factors, including biology, culture, psychology and our environment. For example, our genes can influence our taste preferences and hunger levels, our cultural background can shape our attitudes towards food and eating, and the food environment in which we live can impact our food choices, our eating habits and, consequently, our health outcomes.

Our food environment includes things like the types of food available to us, how easy it is to get them, their cost and the way they are marketed, as well as social and cultural influences. According to the findings of a 2008 study published in the *American Journal of Preventive Medicine*, "Low-income neighbourhoods often lack access to affordable and nutritious food options, leading to disparities in dietary quality and health outcomes among socioeconomically disadvantaged populations."

We can see from all this that food is therefore so much more than just what we put in our mouths. It's a complex interplay between nutrition, emotions and social interactions. And our relationship with it is deeply rooted in our emotional landscape, starting from a young age, where food becomes intertwined with feelings and social situations, such as joy, sadness, celebration, loneliness and anger. Unfortunately, this emotional connection to food can be ingrained in us before we even have control over our own diets, as it's influenced by the choices that our parents or carers make for us.

Just like my mum, I've spent most of my life trapped in a cycle of yo-yo dieting; when my husband Matt and I moved from our flat into our house six years ago, I found eight Slimming World books in the bottom drawer of our kitchen. Eight!

I realised quite some time ago that the reason Slimming World wasn't ever going to be sustainable for me was because, at the core of it, it didn't address the *emotional* reasons why I overeat. As human beings, we are wired to seek pleasure and avoid pain. And eating is no exception. When we experience the discomfort of hunger, we seek pleasure in the form of food. However, when our emotions get involved, we can also begin to avoid other forms of pain related to emotions, and turn to food or drink for comfort, even when we're not necessarily hungry.

This tendency to use food as a coping mechanism for emotional distress can lead to a problematic relationship with food, especially when it comes to certain types of food that trigger the reward centres in our brains. As a result, we can find ourselves caught in a vicious cycle, seeking out these foods for pleasure even when we know they may not be in our best interest in the long term.

EMOTIONAL AND DISORDERED EATING

Emotional eating is extremely common. It's something I've grappled with for years. However, it's when it becomes the primary way to cope with emotions that it can cause issues for us and develop into disordered eating.

I won't go into this in huge detail, but in short, disordered eating is a broad term used to describe irregular eating behaviours that, although not classified as a specific eating disorder, can still have a negative impact on our physical and mental health. These behaviours can include restricting food intake, binge-eating, purging and other forms of compulsive eating habits.

One of the most common forms of disordered eating is binge-eating, which is characterised by eating a large amount of food in a short period of time and feeling a lack of control. This is often followed by feelings of guilt, shame and anxiety. According to a study published in the *Journal of Eating Disorders* (2003), binge-eating is the most common eating disorder in the United States.

Binge-eating is sometimes caused by emotional stress, boredom or anxiety – or a mixture of all three. The National Eating Disorders Association says 50 to 75% of individuals with binge-eating disorder have a history of depression, and many may also have anxiety disorders or substance use disorders. It's also very common for people who have gone through traumatic experiences, like sexual abuse or domestic violence, to develop binge-eating disorder.

In addition to binge-eating disorder, there are several other types of eating disorders that can affect individuals. Here are some common examples:

- **Anorexia nervosa:** This is characterised by an intense fear of gaining weight and a distorted body image. Individuals often severely restrict their food intake, leading to significant weight loss and potential health complications.
- **Bulimia nervosa:** This involves recurrent episodes of binge-eating followed by compensatory behaviours such as self-induced vomiting, excessive exercise or the misuse of laxatives or diuretics.
- **Orthorexia nervosa:** This is not officially recognised as a diagnosable eating disorder, but refers to an obsession with healthy eating and an extreme fixation on consuming only "pure" or "clean" foods.

If you find you are feeling obsessed, excessively guilty or out of control about your eating habits, and you are experiencing physical or emotional distress as a result, it may be a sign that you need to seek professional help, whether from a doctor or mental health professional. There are some resources at the back of this book to help you with this.

AN INTRODUCTION TO "INTUITIVE EATING"

If, like me, you'd like to have a healthier relationship with food, WITHOUT food obsession and dieting, there's an alternative that could help you: a non-diet approach to health and wellness, called "intuitive eating", which has gained popularity in recent years.

The term "intuitive eating" was coined in the 1990s by California-based dieticians Evelyn Tribole and Elyse Resch. Having seen so many of their clients yo-yo dieting and following quick-fix diet plans that always ended in failure, they were inspired to create an evidence-based approach to eating that encourages individuals to listen to their body in relation to what, when and how much to eat. I discovered the concept after reading their book by the same name, *Intuitive Eating*, which I highly recommend.

Tribole and Resch describe intuitive eating as a "personalised approach to making peace with food". The goal is not to lose weight, but rather to cultivate a healthy relationship with food, your body and yourself.

One of the key principles is to reject the diet mentality. This means saying goodbye to quick-fix diets, fad diets and the idea that there are "good" and "bad" foods. Instead, it promotes the idea that all foods can fit into a healthy diet, as long as they're enjoyed in moderation.

Another important aspect of intuitive eating is the idea of "honouring your hunger". This means paying attention to physical hunger cues, such as an empty stomach or lightheadedness, by eating when you're hungry. It also involves listening to your body's fullness cues, such as feeling satisfied or bloated, by stopping when you're comfortably full.

Intuitive eating also encourages us to challenge the internal voices that tell us what we should or shouldn't eat, i.e. our internal "food police". This means letting go of internalised "food rules" and allowing ourselves to eat what we want, when we want it, without guilt or shame.

In addition to challenging "food rules", it encourages you to become more mindful when eating. This means paying attention to the taste, texture and smell of food, as well as being aware of how it makes you feel. Mindful eating helps you to enjoy your food more, and also to become more in tune with your body's natural hunger and fullness cues.

One of the biggest benefits of intuitive eating is the positive impact it can have on mental health. By letting go of the diet mentality and food guilt, you can reduce the stress and anxiety surrounding food, and improve overall self-esteem and body image.

More than 100 academic studies have been done on intuitive eating, including a 2021 meta-analysis that found that the method was positively linked to participants' body image, self-esteem and psychological wellbeing. And while the approach isn't promising better physical health metrics per se, some preliminary studies link intuitive eating to improved blood sugar and cholesterol levels, and less likelihood of developing chronic health conditions such as heart disease and type 2 diabetes, as well as encouraging a more stable weight and a healthier relationship with food.

WHY HAS INTUITIVE EATING BECOME SO POPULAR?

One reason is that it offers a refreshing alternative to traditional diets that focus on weight loss and restriction, instead promoting the idea that you can be healthy and happy at every size, and that food should not be a source of stress or guilt. Another reason for the popularity of intuitive eating is its holistic approach to health in that it takes into account not just physical health, but also mental and emotional wellbeing.

The 10 principles of intuitive eating are:

1. Reject the diet mentality

Diets encourage restriction in some form (whether it's certain foods or certain times to eat), impose rules around foods that are usually not sustainable, and often result in the rules and restrictions being broken (such as by overeating).

One of the reasons we get hooked into diets is because they provide us with a structure and security that if we just follow X number of rules, we'll achieve our weight-loss goals. Unfortunately, this approach can make us begin to think that we *need* these rules and that, without them, we would be powerless to choose well around food for ourselves. As a result of this, many people begin to believe that they are unable to make wise choices and unable to manage without a diet.

When you begin to "reject the diet mentality", and all the diet rules, you effectively have to relearn how to make choices about food for yourself. And relearn that you *can* have power and control over your own choices.

It's then time to throw out the diet books and magazine articles that offer you false hope of losing weight quickly and easily, and instead spend your time working on accepting your body and focusing on things that will bring positivity to your life.

2. Honour your hunger

A big part of intuitive eating is knowing not to view hunger as your enemy, but instead to view it as a useful message or "sign" from your body. The trick is therefore to learn to listen and respond to your early "signs" of hunger by feeding your body. Otherwise, if you let yourself get excessively hungry, you'll be likely to overeat.

For some people, honouring their hunger may mean eating frequently throughout the day; for some it may mean having several large meals a day; for others, it may mean learning to just respond to the physical sensations of hunger as they happen, such as a growling stomach or low energy levels, by eating something nourishing.

3. Make peace with food

The concept of making peace with food is not about mindlessly indulging in junk food all day long. Rather, it's about allowing ourselves to enjoy all foods in moderation and without judgement. When we allow ourselves to eat a wide variety of foods, we're less likely to feel deprived or restricted, which can help us make healthier choices in the long run.

Tribole and Resch – the creators of intuitive eating – say: "Call a truce; stop the food fight! Give yourself unconditional permission to eat. If you tell yourself that you can't or shouldn't have a particular food, it can lead to intense feelings of deprivation that build into uncontrollable cravings and, often, bingeing. When you finally 'give in' to your forbidden foods, eating will be experienced with such intensity, it usually results in Last Supper overeating and overwhelming guilt."

At first you may fear that by giving yourself unconditional permission to eat, you won't be able to stop eating "forbidden" foods, but because all foods are now "allowed", the urgency to have them will get less with time.

4. Challenge our internal "food police"

The way we think, and talk, about food and eating habits tends to be heavily influenced by diet culture, which, as we've seen throughout this book, encourages the labelling of certain foods as "good", "bad" or sometimes "naughty". We might not realise how frequently we use labels like this in how we talk to ourselves about our food choices or in our interactions with family and friends. We might quite often, for example, say things like "I've been good today" or "I was bad and ate a cookie". When we do this, it's our internal "food police" at work.

It's often the case that foods labelled as "bad" by our internal food police are high in sugars, carbs or caffeine content, while foods labelled as "good" are low-fat, low-carb and/or low-calorie. We may even use terms like "boring" and "sensible", and "goodies" and "treats" to classify "good" and "bad" foods – and to acknowledge which ones are "allowed" or not.

However, we can work on changing this mindset simply by being mindful of our thoughts and our language in order to let go of these labels. The first step is simply to start noticing how often we use such terms and then gently reminding ourselves to avoid them, even if it's just in our own minds at first.

As you know by now, food is not good or bad, and you are not good or bad for what you eat or don't eat. So, keep challenging any food-police thoughts that tell you otherwise.

5. Discover the satisfaction factor

Eating should be enjoyable. So, the "satisfaction factor" in intuitive eating is about finding pleasure and joy in the foods we eat. This means choosing foods that we genuinely enjoy, and taking the time to savour them. When we find satisfaction in our food, we're less likely to feel unsatisfied after we eat, which means we are less likely to overeat or get cravings.

It's important to remember that all foods have value in different ways. It's also important to remember that you are never obligated to "finish your plate", even if this was instilled in you growing up. How many times have we tucked into a dinner or dessert only to discover that it's mediocre at best – yet still kept eating? Becoming an "intuitive eater" means leaving any food that you're not enjoying and really savouring the food that you *are* enjoying.

It also means not eating while distracted. A 2011 study by Oldham-Cooper et al. divided a group of people into two halves. One half ate while playing an online game of solitaire, while the other had no distractions at all. The distracted people ate faster, couldn't remember what they ate, ate more snacks and reported feeling significantly less full. Try to remember this the next time that you eat sitting on your sofa watching television or scrolling your phone, and use it as a prompt to turn off the telly or put down your phone.

6. Feel your fullness

Just as your body "tells" you when it's hungry, it also "tells" you when it's full. So, it's important to learn to recognise, and listen for, the signals of when you feel you've had enough, i.e. the signs of comfortable fullness. The trick to this is to eat slowly and mindfully and, as you do so, check in with yourself to see how the food tastes and how hungry or full you are feeling at any stage.

According to Tribole and Resch, respecting your fullness really hinges on giving yourself unconditional permission to eat (Principle 3: make peace with food). This means giving yourself the time to savour your meals without guilt or judgment, and then to honour your level of fullness either by refusing a second helping if that's what you need *or* by enjoying another plate.

The pair also recommend avoiding filling up on what they call "air foods", which clog up our tummies but offer little sustenance as they are so low in calories. Think things like popcorn, rice cakes, celery sticks and Diet Coke.

7. Treat your emotions with kindness

Food is not just something that we put in our mouths (and stomachs)! It's also a way in which we celebrate, commiserate and/or show love and affection. For example, we often go out for a meal to celebrate birthdays, and we comfort ourselves with things like ice cream after a break-up. In a way, eating could be viewed as one of the most emotionally laden experiences that we have in our lives – one that starts from the very day we're born, when we're offered our mother's breast (or a bottle), to stop us crying …

Food is comfort. It's reward. It's love. It's a friend. To be honest, throughout some periods of my life, food has felt like my only friend. So, how do we separate biological hunger from emotional hunger? One way to start is by paying attention to when we feel we're turning to food for emotional comfort. Maybe it's when we're feeling overwhelmed, anxious or bored, for example. Once we can start to recognise these triggers, we'll be able to begin to explore *alternative* ways to soothe ourselves.

We may not have been taught, growing up, how to soothe ourselves in ways that don't involve food, so it's important to *learn* new techniques. You could, for example, try journalling, meditation, therapy or a creative activity like painting or sewing, instead of reaching for more chocolate, biscuits, crisps or whatever else. By learning to soothe ourselves in different ways, we can break the cycle of turning to food for emotional comfort and develop a healthier relationship with both food and our emotions.

Note: if you find yourself eating a lot of food without really enjoying it, just to end up feeling lethargic or even exhausted, it might be helpful to think about talking to an eating disorder specialist or psychotherapist.

8. Respect your body

This means recognising that your worth as a person is not determined by your weight or appearance. When we respect our bodies, we're more likely to make choices that support both our physical and emotional wellbeing. So, for example, rather than criticising your body for how it looks and what you perceive is wrong with it, recognise it as capable, just as it is.

Just as a person with size 9 feet wouldn't expect to squeeze into a size 6, it is equally futile to have a similar expectation when it comes to your body size. Accept your genetic blueprint instead of constantly trying to fight it. And ditch the idea that you're the size you are because you're lacking in willpower, while you're at it.

No doctor would ever suggest that a patient "will" their blood pressure to a normal level, so why should we be able to "will" ourselves thin?! The idea of willpower doesn't belong in the intuitive eating approach, as the whole idea is to respect and *listen to* your personal signals and hunger cues, rather than trying to constantly counteract them.

9. Movement – feel the difference

As we discussed in the last chapter, it's important to find ways to move your body that you enjoy, and to shift the focus of any movement or exercise that you do from losing weight to how you want to *feel*, for example, energised and strong.

It's also vital to understand that you don't need to "earn" food in any way. For example, you don't need to do a tough workout before you're allowed to indulge in a tasty treat, as it's really important to separate our exercise habits from our eating habits. They're two completely different things, so one doesn't need to affect the other.

10. Honour your health with gentle nutrition

If we want to have a healthier relationship with food, we know by now that it's essential to shift our focus from our weight to our overall health and wellbeing. Given that our bodies require "fuel" to have the energy to function, move and maintain good health, it's vital to make wise and gentle choices about what foods we consume. This involves:

- Allowing yourself to eat any food, with no restrictions or limitations
- Giving yourself permission to eat foods that you may have previously labelled as "bad"
- Eating to fuel your body and provide it with the energy it needs
- Trusting your hunger cues and recognising that what works for you may be different from what works for someone else
- Learning that eating at any time of day is OK if your body needs it
- Educating yourself about eating in balance and moderation.

INTUITIVE EATING IS NEITHER A QUICK FIX NOR A CURE-ALL

While intuitive eating can be a really helpful tool for some people, and life-changing for others, it's important to recognise that, like most things, it has its limitations.

One issue is that the approach assumes everyone has equal access to a variety of foods and the ability to listen to their body's signals. However, a lot of people struggle with food poverty and a lot of people have a history of disordered eating that affects their relationship with food, and therefore their natural capacity to recognise their own body's signals. If you fall into either, or both, of these categories, it may mean that intuitive eating isn't for you.

Moreover, intuitive eating is a process that requires a lot of self-reflection and patience. It involves challenging internalised beliefs about, and attitudes towards, food and your body that can be taxing and may require the help of a qualified professional. As such, it's certainly not a "quick fix" or a way to lose weight without effort.

Another misconception about intuitive eating is that it's a license to eat whatever you want, whenever you want – which is not the case.

While I don't think that the approach has been life-changing for me, it has certainly helped me and I really like the freedom and flexibility that it offers, as well as the philosophy behind it.

I also really like the fact that while the creators, Tribole and Resch, sell their books and do trainings for other health professionals, their method has no marketable products or services, such as meal plans, nutritional shakes or branded frozen dinners! Instead, you can read all about the intuitive eating approach online for free, including all the important principles that make it possible to practise on your own.

One study published in the *Journal of Counseling Psychology* in 2006 found that intuitive eating was associated with higher levels of body appreciation and lower levels of body shame among women. Another more recent study published in the *Journal of Nutrition Education and Behavior* in 2021 found that women who practised intuitive eating had a lower risk of disordered eating behaviours, such as binge-eating and purging. That's not to say, of course, that it is by any means a guaranteed way to "fix" disordered eating or your relationship with your body, but it's definitely an approach worth exploring.

I, for one, can say that it's certainly been a much better alternative for me than being in the prison of yo-yo dieting that I had been in for so long before I found this.

There are resources at the end of the book if you'd like to explore intuitive eating further, or if you'd like information about getting help from a specialist.

YOU'RE DOING GREAT

I want to end this chapter by recognising that the journey towards a healthier relationship with food is not linear, nor is it without its challenges. It involves cultivating a sense of mindfulness and compassion towards ourselves and our bodies – something that diet culture has never encouraged.

So, remember, every small step counts. Whether it's eating without guilt, learning to listen to your body's signals, or practising more self-care, it's important to embrace your unique journey, wherever you are on it, and recognise that progress, not perfection, is key.

Above all, be kind to yourself and know deep down that your life's purpose is not to permanently be on a diet.

SELF-EMPOWERMENT TASK

Take a little time out for yourself and think about the history of your relationship with food. See if you can jot down any memories that stand out from different stages of your life, starting from when you were young, in terms of how you have felt about food at different times. Think about any key events that *shaped* how you feel about it.

Do you see any patterns emerging? And can you see how these things may still be impacting you?

12

Finding your style
Building confidence and feeling fabulous

I couldn't write this book without mentioning style and fashion, because it's been a really big part of my journey towards self-acceptance. While talking about clothes might seem superficial, I truly believe it can be a key part of feeling confident and being unapologetically you. Finding your personal style can do wonders for your self-esteem, as can questioning the hard-and-fast fashion "rules" of what women can and can't wear.

For years I grew up listening to people like Trinny and Susannah (British fashion advisors and TV presenters) telling me I couldn't wear stripes (or white, or skinny jeans, or turtlenecks, or bold patterns or anything that wasn't A-line). In one episode of their makeover TV series (which I happened to stumble across recently on TikTok), the pair are seen ripping a woman to shreds about her muffin top, poor posture, terrible hair and bad skin. It really gave me the ick.

I'm here to tell you that you don't need to pay attention to fashion rules, and that you don't need to wear clothes just because they're "flattering".

Fashion should be FUN. So let's make it fun and get playful with our wardrobes.

HOW I FOUND MY PERSONAL STYLE

I have always loved fashion, but it's fair to say fashion hasn't always loved me. Growing up fat and with little money meant that, for the most part, I had to wear just whatever I could get my hands on that would fit on my body. And that had a huge impact on my self-esteem.

I pretty much always wore clothes that were a bit too small or didn't suit me – partly because I think I was in denial about my size, but also because, shock horror, I just wanted to wear what everyone else my age was wearing. I desperately wanted to go into Jane Norman and Tammy Girl and Topshop, and wear all the things my friends could. But, instead, I was more often than not relegated to the accessories section in such shops (I definitely blame this for my ongoing obsession with bags and scarves, given that I didn't have to worry about whether these would "fit" me or not!). I even remember trying on clothes in Topshop, knowing they wouldn't fit, just so I didn't seem like a complete loser to my friends, and then making up some excuse to the sales assistant about the colour not being right.

For most of my teenage years, I wore black – for fear of standing out more than I already did. In my 20s, I did feel a bit more confident with my style, but, as a UK size 22 (US size 18), I was still extremely limited with what I could buy. I remember being a student and raiding the supermarkets for clothes because nothing else would really fit me. For the majority of my teenage years into early adulthood, I shopped solely in Dorothy Perkins; there's nothing wrong with Dorothy Perkins, of course, but a girl likes to have options.

I refused to shop in plus-size-only stores because the options there were so limited. It felt like the only thing they had to offer me were cold-shoulder tops with butterflies on, or shapeless tunics with diamantés applied (maybe an Eiffel Tower if I was lucky) all over them.

It really wasn't until I was about 24 that things changed. ASOS launched its Curve range, and, for the first time in my life, I had access to on-trend clothes in my size. I was just out of university so I still didn't have a lot of money, but what I saved from my job working in a pub I splurged on anything and everything I could. Finally, I could wear clothes that fitted both my body and my personality, instead of "making do". It really was a game-changer.

Fast forward a few years, and I now have a wardrobe full of colourful clothes that fit me and that I love. And it's made the world of difference to how I feel about fashion.

To get to this point, though, I had to experiment a lot, trying things that I didn't think would suit me, as well as things that I knew would. For example, I always wore jeans growing up but, through my experimentation, I discovered a huge love for dresses, and that really helped me feel feminine after years of feeling anything but. I also experimented a lot with colour and – this is an important one – I started to ignore the sizes on the labels.

Through my experimentation, I also realised quite some time ago that women's sizing is bullshit. Clothing manufacturers these days often use what is called "vanity sizing", which means that they label clothes with sizes smaller than the actual cut of the items. Retailers seem to think that being able to fit into a smaller size will make us feel better about ourselves, which will make us more likely to buy from them (and keep buying from them!).

The rise of so-called vanity sizing has rendered most labels meaningless. I have things in my wardrobe now that are everything from a UK size 22 (US size 18) to a UK size 32 (US size 28). So, please don't let an arbitrary number on a label determine how you feel about yourself or your happiness. Clothing should fit *us*, not the other way around.

WHAT WE DO WANT FROM RETAILERS

I know it isn't always easy finding clothes (especially if you're plus size, tall, short, disabled, big-chested, small-chested … or if you have big hips, shoulders or whatever else …).

I think a lot of brands fall down when it comes to being inclusive. I can't tell you the amount of times I've seen something I love and want to buy, only to find that it stops at a UK size 20 (US size 16). *Or* that it's available in plus size but some genius has decided to re-tailor it into a sack, because god forbid a woman over a UK size 20 wants to wear something fitted.

It's also really hard when you're limited to buying clothes online, because many brands still use smaller models, which means you can't see what it looks like on a bigger person. Is being able to go into a physical store and buy clothes in our size too much to ask? Is our money not as good as everyone else's?

As I briefly mentioned back in Chapter 4, I'd also like to encourage brands to have some fat perspective in their buying teams, or at the very least to engage with the plus-size community. For some reason, many current buyers seem to think we want everything to be a little bit "jazzy". God forbid we'd want to wear a plain black T-shirt. No, it has to have holes cut out of the arms, tassels and maybe even the words "rock chick" emblazoned over it for good measure.

While plus-size shopping is definitely so much better than it used to be, we'd love to see brands become more inclusive and not just promise they're "working on it". We want to see more clothes modelled on different body types, so we can really get an idea of what they'd actually look like on us. And we'd also love to see brands standardise their sizing and produce accurate size charts, to take the guesswork (and therefore some of the size stress) out of our shopping sessions.

STYLE TIPS

If you're in a bit of a style rut and looking to change up your wardrobe, here are a few tips for you:

Get rid of your "failure" dress

A failure dress is that one dress (or it could be a top, or a pair of jeans) that's way too small but you've kept for when you get down to your "goal weight". Please, do yourself a favour and get rid of this. You will never feel at home in a body that you view as "temporary". And you deserve both to feel at home in your body and to feel joy and excitement (not guilt and shame) when you open your wardrobe. What's more, even if you did "lose the weight" so that the dress finally fitted you, the chances are that you may not like it anymore anyway!

My failure dress was a beautiful blue tea dress from Debenhams in a UK size 14 (US size 10). I got it in the sale for a bargain price and even though I could barely get it on, I bought it and kept it for years. It was beautifully made, lined and had little white daisies on it. I kept it for when I was "slimmer" – for Laura 2.0. But every time I saw it in my wardrobe, it was a reminder of an arbitrary goal that I'd "failed" to achieve, and it made me feel shitty.

After holding onto it for about eight years, I finally decided to give it to charity, and, do you know, it was one of the best things I did for myself. It created space in my wardrobe for clothes that did fit and made me feel freer.

Consider what you actually *like*, not what's in your size

Don't get me wrong, I love floral midi-dresses as much as the next fat bird, but lately I've been questioning whether I *actually* like them, or whether I wear them because there's just so many of them available in my size.

In their book *Happy Fat*, comedian Sofie Hagan has an interesting theory about fat women wearing floral dresses as a sort of apology. They say: "I wear floral dresses as an apology for my existence, as if to say: 'I'm sorry I'm taking up space, I'm sorry I'm not the kind of person you want me to be, but look, at least I'm pretty.'"

If you love a floral midi, wear one. But next time you're shopping, really think about your style. Is it minimalist, or bold, or daring? Do you like colour or prefer more neutral tones? Do you enjoy wearing midi and maxi dresses, or would you like to show a bit more leg? Get experimenting and think about what you like, with no fear of what other people think.

Fuck "flattering"

Trinny and Susannah would have us believe that the entire point of clothes is for them to flatter our body shape and size. Personally, I think flattering can mean wearing styles and colours that suit your personality or skin tone, just as much as your body shape and size. But, for the most part, it's used as a way of saying something makes us look smaller than we are.

I've come to the conclusion that I'm fat whether I wear a "slimming" little black dress or a hot pink bodycon number. So, given a combination of this and the fact that someone is likely to judge me for my size or shape no matter what I wear, fuck "flattering"!

Let's wear what we want and what makes us feel good.

Find your style hero(es)

I'd probably describe my style as "Fat Holly Willoughby". I love her feminine, minimalist style and will often look at what she's wearing to see if I can find things that are similar in my size.

If you're not sure about your own personal style, take some time out to research and gather together visual inspiration for looks that you like, and put together a mood board of your favourites, whether on Instagram, Pinterest or elsewhere.

Last but not least, don't be afraid to push yourself out of your comfort zone and experiment. You can rock a grungy outfit one day and a floral dress the next. There are no rules.

Use colour as a form of expression

I know this may sound harsh, but wearing *only* black doesn't make you look slimmer, it just makes you look boring.

Working bolder hues such as bright pink or blue into your wardrobe is a great way to showcase your personality and personal style AND make you feel good.

There's been a huge uptick in "dopamine dressing" recently – which, if you haven't heard of it, is a way to dress yourself happy by utilising colour. It not only affects *your* mood, but also that of those around you. So, if you want to, ditch the dull and start embracing colour. The bolder and brighter the better.

221

If it feels daunting, start small by going for a pop of colour via just your accessories.

Don't save your nice clothes for best

Don't wait for an occasion to wear something you love. Even if it means wearing it to the supermarket, who cares? Get your money's worth out of your purchases by getting out in your best gear.

By keeping something "for best", you're telling yourself you're not good enough as you are *now* to wear it.

On the contrary, the philosophy of *not* saving your clothes for best is a declaration of self-love and empowerment. It's a reminder that you deserve to feel your best every single day, not just on rare occasions. Whether it's a sparkling sequined top or a pair of killer heels that make your heart sing, these pieces hold the power to boost your confidence and elevate your mood, no matter where you're headed.

Bin the shapewear (but do invest in good underwear)

Don't tell anyone, but I once nearly shit myself at a friend's wedding because I was wearing the most awful Spanx that were two sizes too small and killing me!

Please don't make the same mistake I did. They just make you look like a sausage and you'll feel miserable.

Do, however, invest in some really good underwear. We've all got knickers in our drawer with holes in (or at least I know I do) and dedicated period pants. But it's also good to invest in some decent, supportive, comfortable, quality underwear that doesn't roll down or cut you in half. And – if you want – make sure you have some in your wardrobe that make you feel super sexy, too. It doesn't have to be expensive; supermarkets often do some great lingerie options these days.

If you do nothing else when it comes to underwear, be sure to at least get a proper bra fitting. It's estimated around 80% of women are wearing the wrong size bra. And having the proper support for your bazookas will make the world of difference in how you feel and how your clothes sit on you.

Ditch the trends

Trends can be great if you're in your early 20s or have a ton of disposable income. But for me, leaning into trends via the occasional item here and there is enough these days; as, for the most part, my wardrobe is full of timeless pieces that I can wear again and again.

My advice is therefore to shop with intention. Look at what's missing from your wardrobe and try to find that in order to create a really effective capsule wardrobe. As part of this, be sure to choose colours that complement your skin tone and lines that complement your shape, as well as garments that generally suit your personality, of course!

Comfort is king

This is arguably the most important piece of advice I can give you: avoid clothes that dig in, fall down or generally make you feel uncomfortable. If you're comfortable, you'll likely feel more confident, and confidence is key.

If you feel confident in something, I guarantee you'll wear it better. So often we're told by the body-positive police that wearing a bikini is the epitome of body confidence – "just wear the damn bikini". But I don't think this is always true. Sure, it's great to feel the sun on your belly when you feel comfortable doing so, but sometimes showing up comfortably is worth more than proving anything.

It's not about what you wear. It's about being there in whatever you feel comfortable in. That's the win. That's the point.

SELF-EMPOWERMENT TASK

Take a little time for yourself and sort out your wardrobe. I promise you'll feel better for it. Get absolutely everything out and plonk it on your bed. And yes, I mean absolutely everything … knickers, bras, pyjamas and all. We're going full Marie Kondo here.

Try everything on and ask yourself: "Does it fit me? Does it make me feel good – ideally great?" If the answer is yes, pop it back in your wardrobe, ideally categorised by type. If the answer is no, sell it or donate it. (SmartWorks is an amazing UK-based charity which helps women get back on their feet and into work; alternatively, if you're based elsewhere, ask around or look up reputable charities in your area and decide which one(s) you'd like to support.)

You should end up with a wardrobe of clothes that you know will both fit and make you feel fabulous. And that means saying goodbye to the wardrobe meltdowns we've all had before going on a night out.

13

Dating and relationships

You deserve to be loved, just as you are

When you're plus size (or if your appearance doesn't conform to mainstream beauty standards in other ways), dating can seem fraught with even more challenges than otherwise. It's not a level playing field, and there's no point pretending it is.

My love life was pretty much non-existent until I started online dating around the age of 22 (back when it was still considered a bit weird).

Until that point, I'd had a couple of flings with people at university, but I didn't really have any confidence with dating, sex or relationships because I genuinely thought I was too fat to find love. I didn't even have my first orgasm until I was 24.

But, bored and lonely in my little flat one night, I decided to log onto one of the OG dating sites, Plenty Of Fish, and see what it was all about. I filled out my profile and uploaded the most flattering picture I could find … with great lighting, perfect hair, the perfect pout, and almost enough make-up for RuPaul to raise an eyebrow.

The first ever message I got was from someone who referred to me as a BBW (big beautiful woman). It was a phrase that I'd never even heard of before, but one that I'd soon come to know very well.

"Hey BBW, looking for fun?" the message said.

Soon, another one popped up in my inbox: "I'm *really* into BBWs."

And then another: "Talk to me, BBW."

All of the messages were overtly sexual and all of them were about my body. Don't get me wrong, I expected to get explicit photos and unwanted advances. But I was taken aback by the abundance of messages carrying an undertone of entitlement. There was an assumption that my body was somehow theirs for the taking purely because of the size of it.

How did I go from feeling completely de-sexualised by society to suddenly being fetishised in abundance by creepy men online? The whole thing was a minefield and, to be honest, it made me feel a bit dirty (and not in a good way).

Like many of us, all I wanted was to be loved for who I was – not *because* of my body and not *in spite of* it. Was that too much to ask?

I did eventually find love (on that very same dating site, would you believe?) and am now happily married. But it wasn't easy getting there.

While I want to stress that not all fat people have lived through sex and relationship horror stories, here's what many of us have faced in the search for love:

- Being hypersexualised or even fetishised
- Being kept a secret

- Feelings being one-sided
- Being more concerned with being liked than checking in to see how *we* feel about the person
- Them only wanting sex
- Being made to feel like we should be grateful

As well as bringing to light what so many of us have to put up with in the quest for love, in this chapter I also want to share my top tips for dating when you're plus size, with the help of relationships expert and author of *The Selfish Romantic,* Michelle Elman.

If you're *not* single, I hope you might find that some of the suggestions in the pages that follow will help if you're struggling with any insecurities in an existing relationship.

We'll be looking at the importance of *non*-romantic love, too.

THE WORLD OF PLUS-SIZE DATING

Let's dive for a moment into some of the intricacies of online dating, from agonising over what photos to upload to your profile to the fear of rejection …

What photos to use?

You might not like this, but it's time to upload a full-length photo. Maybe two. A selfie from your favourite angle is lovely – and I know I definitely filled my profiles with them too – but we know those angles show us in a very flattering light. You need to show your potential dates what you really look like, in full.

Personally, I think it's also good to show potential matches *who* you are, not just what you look like. So why not share photos of you doing things you love, whether that's out with your friends, on holiday, in nature, reading a book, eating food, cycling, baking, etc.?

Fetishisation or attraction?

It's completely understandable that we're wary of people's intentions, given the society we live in and the horror stories we've all heard about "hogging" or "pulling a pig", which is when men are dared to sleep with a fat woman by their friends.

But, while it's important to be wary of people who just want to fetishise us or use us, we also need to reject the notion that attraction to someone who is fat is a fetish. Not everyone who's into fat women is automatically fetishising them. Some people just prefer bigger women, and that's OK. Attraction is a personal thing and it's all about individual preferences.

When it becomes a problem is when we're reduced to just our bodies. That's when attraction crosses over into fetishisation territory, and that's when we need to be careful.

Getting over the fear of rejection

With your heart on the line, it can feel like your whole world has crumbled around you if you happen to be rejected by someone. However, it's important to remember that rejection is a completely normal part of dating for *everyone*. Not every person you meet will find you attractive or a compatible match, and that's OK. It's not a reflection of your worth. You won't find every person *you* meet attractive or a compatible match either.

"A big way of saving yourself from the hurt of rejection is reframing it," says Elman. "Most of the time they're not rejecting you, they're rejecting your profile. So if they don't know you, they can't reject you. A lot of the time we increase the hurt that we experience because we're tracking the rejection. Realising and accepting that not everyone is going to fancy you, just like you don't fancy everyone, can help shift your mindset. Just because someone doesn't fancy you, it doesn't mean you're unfanciable or unworthy."

The same applies to ghosting (when someone cuts off communication without explanation). If someone ghosts you, it's not a reflection on you, but a sign that they're either not a good fit for you or that they're not emotionally available. And who wants that?

"If someone chooses to ghost rather than communicate, it's an indicator that they struggle with communication in general," explains Elman. "And that's the same kind of person who, when in a relationship, is going to be silent rather than actually tell you they're angry with you. That's the kind of person who's just going to stop texting every time you get into a fight, rather than actually communicating through the difficult conversations. Someone ghosting is showing you that up front and will save you heartache in the long run. It's better to find out early so you can weed that person out and move on."

Elman also stresses the importance of not assuming someone is ghosting because of our weight or physical appearance.

"We cannot read someone's mind; implicit in ghosting is the fact there is no explanation, so do not assume a narrative to hurt yourself more. So often we jump to the worst possible conclusion in our minds and take other people's behaviour personally. In reality, if someone ghosts, they've likely ghosted before and they likely will ghost again. It's not personal to you and it's not a reflection of your worth."

Not settling for second best

It's completely normal to make assumptions about what other people view as attractive or unattractive. As we discussed back in Chapter 3, societal beauty standards have often focused on a narrow range of traits, such as specific body types, skin tones or facial features. But please remember what I've been saying throughout this entire book: your outward appearance is just one piece of the whole beautiful puzzle (and often the least interesting part).

Don't match with people you think are only half good enough for you, and never assume that someone is "out of your league".

What changed things for me when I was dating was asking myself if I actually liked the person I was with. At first, I had never actually stopped to ask myself that question before because I was so focused on whether or not they liked me.

I wish I'd realised sooner the importance of not settling for second best (or even third best at times) just because I was scared of being on my own (or scared that there would be no one else out there for me).

It's hard to feel confident about being on your own when society places so much value on being in a relationship. It often feels like the biggest achievement you can make in your life is to be "settled down" with someone and married with 2.4 children.

But being single is not a problem to be fixed, and it's far better to be single than to be in a relationship that's "wrong". In fact, Elman says that actively choosing to be single can be a valuable learning experience.

She notes: "Although often well meaning, when people say things like, 'How are you still single?', it implies that no one would actually *choose* to be single. And actually, you can learn so much in the time you're on your own. I learned that I needed to get comfortable with being alone, or else I would end up settling. And so I forced myself to spend alone time with myself, scheduling a Friday night to sit alone on my sofa and do small things that I would do if I had a friend or boyfriend over. I also opened my mind to the fact that dating *can* be fun and that it's not all doom and gloom. I really made the most of my eight years of single life and I'm so grateful I did."

TIPS FOR WHEN YOU *ARE* OUT ON A DATE

You've been getting along really well on messages, maybe even on the phone or video calls – and you're preparing to meet up in real life. You're probably shitting yourself about what your date will think of how you look (especially if you didn't include some full-length profile photos). So, here's a run-down of some things to consider …

- **Dress comfortably.** As I mentioned before, comfort is king. Don't feel like you have to dress up to the nines. Just be your authentic self.
- **Don't bring up your weight.** While I think adding a full-length picture to your profile is a good thing for honesty, I also think it's important to avoid bringing up your size or weight (at least too much) when you're in the early stages – to avoid it seeming like it's a big deal. Dating is about forming connections with others based on mutual interests, compatibility and shared values. Your weight is just one aspect of who you are, and the focus should be on building a genuine connection, rather than fixating on physical appearance.
- **Don't be afraid to EAT.** Confidence is key in any dating situation. So, embrace who you are and eat what you want – not what you *think* you should have in this situation.

LET'S TALK ABOUT SEX, BABY

There's so much bloody pressure and stigma around sex, isn't there? I don't know about you, but I definitely grew up in a household where sex wasn't talked about, and it's taken an awful lot of un-learning as an adult to realise that a) it's not something to shy away from and b) it's nothing like we see in porn.

Sex when you're plus size, especially if you're dating, can cause lots of insecurities to bubble to the surface. So, here are some tips for when it comes to sex and body insecurities:

- **STOP FAKING YOUR ORGASMS**. It's not helping them, and it's not helping you. According to a 2017 survey by Durex, only 65% of women having sex with a man have an orgasm, compared to 95% of men having sex with a woman. When you fake it, you're putting their needs above your own. You deserve better.
- **Practise self-pleasure**. God, how I wish someone had told me this when I was younger! There is no shame in masturbation. If you don't know what you like, how can you expect your partner to know? Experiment, buy toys and have fun on your own.
- **Stop hiding your body**. For years I was terrified of trying different positions because I was worried about my body being too big or too "on show". Or I would try and hide my stomach by wearing a T-shirt, or squashing it down with my hands. "Don't be afraid to try new things and don't be afraid to get on top," says sex educator Shakira Scott (also known as Scotty Unfamous). "If he dies, he dies." (Obviously she's joking, but you get the gist!)
- **Communicate your needs**. Scott also says, "I always think it's a bit bizarre how we can be so comfortable putting someone's dick in our mouth, but not tell them what we like and what we don't [like]."

After all, how can they know if what they're doing is good for us or not if we don't ever even let them know?

- **Communicate your fears**. As important as telling your partner what you *like*, is telling them what you're nervous or anxious about. It's often something they've never even thought of. By getting it off your chest, you can talk about it, have things out in the open and move on.
- **Consider keeping the light on**. "All that stuff about leaving the lights off, leaving your shirt on, even leaving your make-up intact because you're worried they might be put off if you remove it – it's actually just making you super aware of your own body," says Elman. "The more you overthink things, the less you're able to connect with your body. And if you're not really in sync with your body, having an orgasm becomes a bit of a challenge because it's all about feeling, not thinking."

I won't lie – there are some things in the list above that I still struggle with. I'm still working on my relationship with sex and intimacy. It's just so easy to overthink things when it comes to intimacy and our bodies.

But, firstly, let's remember that almost *everyone* has insecurities, regardless of their body shape, size and whatever else. So, the person you're with is probably thinking about their own body (or the sex that's about to happen), rather than thinking about, or analysing, *your* body in detail.

Instead of getting stuck in your head, try to focus on the sensations you're experiencing in your body. Pay attention to where your partner is touching you, and really engage with everything happening.

And remember, if you're with someone, it's because they've already made a decision to be with you – you haven't misled or deceived them in any way. So, trust that they find you attractive and enjoy the experience.

Elman agrees: "When it comes to sex, I often hear people worrying about what will happen when they take their top off – like suddenly they'll be seen as 'fat'. First things first, being 'fat' is not the ultimate bedroom nightmare. And second, if you weren't 'fat' before you whipped off that shirt, guess what? The absence of fabric isn't going to magically make you fat. And if you were fat from the start, well, news flash – your partner already knows. So, that moment of revealing? It's not the dramatic plot twist we build it up to be."

WHAT IF MY PARTNER DOESN'T FIND ME SEXUALLY ATTRACTIVE?

This is such a hard one. When things aren't going brilliantly in a relationship, it's all too easy to jump to the conclusion that our partner doesn't find us attractive any more. It's important to remember that levels of sexual desire fluctuate over the course of a lifetime, which means that ebbs and flows are perfectly normal.

A decline in desire is not necessarily an indication of a problem. BUT, if you feel like your partner just isn't showing you as much physical affection or showering you with as many compliments as they used to, then there are a range of ways that you can start to bring that to their attention:

Express your needs without blame

I totally get that it might feel uncomfortable or vulnerable, but it's important to communicate with your partner if you're feeling neglected or rejected. Ask them if they're still feeling physically attracted to you, and, if you can manage it, whether they're feeling happy with your current sex life. Try not to make either accusations or demands; there is validity in both your *and* your partner's desires and preferences.

Be clear about what you want

Don't expect your partner to read your mind. Instead, clearly express what you would like from the relationship. Whether it's more frequent initiation of sex, increased physical affection or occasional compliments, just gently let your partner know. Open communication is key to understanding, and trying to meet, one another's needs.

Initiate sex more often

If you feel your partner isn't instigating sex as much as you'd like them to, take the leap to instigate more sex yourself, and see how they react. It's natural for one person in a relationship to initiate sex more frequently; it doesn't necessarily mean that your partner doesn't want you.

Set clear boundaries

If sex is really important to you, and your partner continuously doesn't make any effort to recognise this and meet your needs, then you may need to consider your options. It can be difficult to end a relationship, especially a long-term one, but it's important to question whether living with someone who doesn't truly acknowledge your needs is worth it.

If you take this decision, it will then be liberating to realise that there are other people who will find you attractive and be willing and able to meet your needs. Elman says: "If your partner is incapable of meeting your needs, then it may be time to find someone who can. Having difficult conversations may be uncomfortable in the short term, but it's worth it for a lifetime of happiness and fulfilment. You deserve to be with someone who values and appreciates you for who you are."

PLATONIC RELATIONSHIPS ARE IMPORTANT, TOO

We all know that relationships are important for our wellbeing. But why is the focus so often placed on romantic ones? What about placing more emphasis on the utmost importance of platonic relationships, too, including having relationships with people who look at least somewhat like you when it comes to body shape and size.

Community can change the way you feel about anything – including your own body. Making friends with people who have shared life experiences, including that of living in a larger body, can bond you and inspire you. Such friends may well be able to provide a safe space to talk about the challenges of navigating a fatphobic world and to share resources when it comes to things like finding clothes that fit, finding open-minded healthcare providers and other such necessities.

Every day, I see incredible friendships form in the community Facebook group that we created on the back of my *Go Love Yourself* podcast. Sometimes it's over little things, like finally finding a belt that fits around your waist, and other times it's bigger stuff, like how to cope with criticism about your weight from a "well-intended" family member.

As we've been exploring in earlier chapters, it can be isolating for those of us in larger bodies. Finding a community of people who share your experiences can provide an incredible source of comfort, validation and joy.

But the benefits of platonic relationships go far beyond just finding people who share your experiences, of course. Friends of all shapes and sizes can help bring more of a sense of belonging, purpose and meaning to our lives. We all have a fundamental need for connection, which means that finding people who accept us for who we are can be incredibly fulfilling.

Platonic relationships can often provide a different kind of support than romantic ones. While romantic relationships can be wonderful, they often come with their own set of specific challenges and expectations. Platonic relationships, on the other hand, can (when they work well), be a source of unconditional love and support, without the pressure of meeting certain "romantic" expectations.

So, how do you find this kind of friendship community? I'd suggest starting by seeking out spaces where you can connect with others who share your experiences. This could be online groups or in-person meetups.

You could look at joining a community related to something you're passionate about, like a choir, an amateur dramatic society, a book club or a Harry Potter games night. There's a new friend out there for everyone. Or you might want to look for events or groups that are centred around body positivity, fat liberation or other such issues that resonate with you.

I'm not proud to admit that I used to be embarrassed of having fat friends. I worried about what people would think or say when they saw two fat people together, and that we'd be even more of a target.

I wish I'd known before how truly incredible it feels to have a safe place to talk about things that only affect plus-size people. It's made me feel much more secure, confident, seen, heard and supported. I don't have to worry about feeling judged when I need more space or when I complain about a seat that's too small. With my fat friends, I can be open about my needs and feelings as a larger woman. And that's magical.

I'd go as far as to say that having friends who understand both the struggles and joys of living in a plus-size body can not only be life-*affirming* but, ultimately, life-*changing*.

DON'T SETTLE – YOU DESERVE ONLY THE BEST

Navigating love and relationships, whether romantic or otherwise, is tricky. But, as we've mentioned a few times throughout the book, it can sometimes feel that, when you're bigger, you have to make up for your body in other ways, like being the funniest or most outgoing person in the room – as if those things will somehow cancel out your appearance. That's really damaging, because it puts pressure on you to be "perfect" in various other aspects of your life.

In reality, there's nothing wrong with your body and you don't have to compensate for anything. You deserve people in your life who love, respect and support you just as you are. So if someone can't see past your body to appreciate the person you are, then they're not worth your time or energy.

"Our bodies are constantly changing and we have no control over that," says Elman. "We could get sick, lose or gain weight, and so on. So we shouldn't want someone to love us just because of our body, which can change at any moment. On the other hand, we also don't want someone to love us *despite* our body, because that implies our body is something to be ashamed of. We are more than just our bodies, so deserve to be loved for who we are as a whole person."

It's definitely not easy, but be kind to yourself and know you deserve only good things when it comes to love and friendships.

And if you *are* looking for love – don't let your insecurities become obstacles, and don't ever settle for less than you deserve.

SELF-EMPOWERMENT TASK

Take a little time out for yourself and have a think about the main relationships in your life – both romantic and platonic. Do they leave you feeling fully seen, heard, accepted, supported, nourished and loved in all ways, including when it comes to your body shape and size?

If so, fantastic. If not, might it be worth seeking out some more like-minded and/or "like-bodied" people – to bring an increased sense of belonging and understanding into your daily life? Are there any groups or communities, whether locally or online, that you could reach out to with this in mind?

14

Breaking the cycle

Overcoming diet culture for a brighter future

As a society, we definitely need to work towards creating a more inclusive and accepting environment for people of all sizes – one in which people's appearances are a non-issue.

In this chapter, we're going to consider – with the help of Molly Forbes – body positivity campaigner, mother of two and author of *Body Happy Kids* – how we can start to break the intergenerational cycle of fatphobia and diet culture that so many of us have been stuck in. Molly is also founding director of The Body Happy Organisation, a social enterprise dedicated to promoting positive body image in children.

As I see it, there are two main ways we can do our bit to stop the cycle from spilling into the next generation: we can be an ally to those in marginalised bodies, and we can be mindful of what we teach to our children. So let's explore each of these more …

HOW TO BE AN ALLY TO FAT PEOPLE

I want to begin by looking at how to be an ally to fat people and why it's so important.

If you're in a fat body yourself, feel free to pass this section to your nearest and dearest, although you might also find it useful yourself. I think sometimes we can be so focused on our own struggles, that we forget about those who are larger than us.

Whatever our size, we need to stop using phrases like "At least I'm not that fat" and "I feel so fat today". While they may seem harmless, what we're actually saying to anyone who is bigger than us is: "I'm doing my very best to not be like you."

As we've been exploring in this book, moving through the world in a fat body is not always easy; discrimination is still a reality for those of us who inhabit the size of body that society tells us "shouldn't" exist.

So, if you don't live in a fat body, or if you're plus size but can still buy clothes in-store and navigate public transport without an issue, how can you step up and fight alongside larger people as a genuine ally?

This is where the subject of acknowledging privilege comes in. I am someone who has privilege because I'm white. Like most privilege, I didn't ask for it and I can't give it away, but I can use it to speak out against injustice whenever I can.

And it's no different with body privilege: the smaller you are, the more body privilege you have; the bigger you are, the less you have. As we covered in Chapter 6, very large people face discrimination in healthcare, getting jobs, when buying clothes, on public transport … the list is endless.

So here are some tips and advice on how to be a better ally to fat people:

1. Do your research
One of the first steps to being a good ally in any space is knuckling down and doing your homework. Carve out time to learn about the pervasiveness of diet culture, and the many ways that it affects all of us, particularly when it comes to the "wellness" movement.

Read up on the "obesity crisis" and the damaging impact of appearance-driven diets. Delve deeper into the body positivity movement. Learn about the significant barriers to adequate healthcare that fat people face. Discover the "size ceiling" that fat people – particularly women – experience in workplaces. Learn about the microaggressions that we fear, or are exhausted by, daily.

2. Acknowledge society's barriers
Numerous studies have shown over the past decade that fat people face significant systemic, structural and institutional barriers. Discrimination against fat people is so endemic, it's difficult for many to acknowledge that it's happening, even among those who are targeted. As we've heard, fat people face greater health risks, are less likely to be hired, work longer hours and are paid less.

One important step towards addressing the discrimination against higher-weight individuals is therefore to fully acknowledge the discriminatory challenges that exist for people living in larger bodies and to help increase awareness about the impact of this.

3. Watch your language and call out others

Be mindful of the words and phrases you use when talking about food, diets and bodies. Assigning moral value to food and bodies is damaging for us all. Check yourself. If you're changing the way you eat, or examining your relationship with your own body, that's fine. But always be mindful about how, or if, you talk about it.

If you hear others saying things like "I'm being good today about what I eat", "I feel so fat today that I can barely move" or "I can't believe she's found love at her size while I can't even get a text back", don't be afraid to challenge them. It can be as simple as phrasing some of their words back to them as a question, such as "What does 'being good' really mean?" or "How can 'fat' be a feeling?" Alternatively, you can be blunt and call them out on how insulting what they're saying feels to you, and that it makes them look like a dick. It's up to you.

4. Don't make assumptions

Never assume that a fat person in your life wants to change their body or that they want advice on it. Many of us are dealing with disordered eating or its fallout. For example, while I personally will never diet again, I can still tell you, from force of habit, the approximate amount of calories that almost any food contains, and I still feel anxious about eating alone in public, given the shame that I associated with eating for so long.

Making assumptions that fat people might want to lose weight, that they are or should be dieting, that they hate their bodies or are uncomfortable with themselves, can therefore be incredibly damaging, perpetuating the shame and self-loathing that fat people are taught to feel.

Whatever your size, we all need to be allies to the most vulnerable, unpack our own feelings about fatness, embrace the uncomfortable and stand up for those who aren't always able to stand up for themselves.

UNDERSTANDING THE INTERGENERATIONAL CYCLE OF DIET CULTURE

Now that we've covered how to be an ally, I want to talk more about breaking the intergenerational cycle of diet culture.

As children, we pick up on, and therefore "learn", many beliefs and values from simply observing our parents' behaviour. Psychologists call this modelling. Modelling can be both positive and negative.

To give a few examples, if your mum – like mine – constantly criticised her weight and her body, and told you that she couldn't eat what everyone else was eating because she needed to fit into her new dress, you learn that women have to look a certain way, and that restricting food helps you do that. If your sister frequently gets complimented on her appearance, and seems popular and happy, it tells you that being beautiful is important, and affects how people treat you. If your dad criticises the breakfast TV presenter for "letting herself go", you learn that men habitually judge a woman's appearance, and that not looking a certain way can lead you to be ridiculed.

Personally, I found growing up in a house consumed by diet talk really tough. Once, in a supermarket, my mum and I saw a woman browsing the cereal aisle when she turned to me and said, "If I ever get that fat, shoot me." I must have only been about 13. I remember scanning this woman from head to toe, analysing every detail of her outfit, every curve of her body. I didn't say anything. I just remember being a bit taken aback and thinking: "Must. Never. Get. That. Fat."

I spent a lot of time watching my mum eat differently to the rest of us growing up, and seeing her self-esteem ebb and flow with every weight loss or gain. Most Sundays she would cook us a roast dinner with all the trimmings. But while we were all tucking into Yorkshire puddings and roast potatoes, she would have plain chicken with boiled potatoes and steamed veg. Gravy was replaced by a small teaspoon of ketchup.

The other thing I noticed growing up was how my dad always praised her for "being good" when it came to her food choices, and how differently he treated her when she was in a smaller body. It was like she was more worthy, more attractive and more loveable when she was smaller.

She told me once, after she'd reached her goal weight on whatever new diet plan she was on, that she called the team leader of the group and asked her when she would start to feel different. Confused, the team leader asked her what she meant. She genuinely thought she would reach her goal weight and that everything would suddenly click into place and she would feel like a happier, more satisfied person. So she was devastated to be told it wouldn't change anything but her body. She'd been sold this lie that her life would be transformed when she hit her goal weight; like a caterpillar turning into a butterfly, or an ugly duckling into a swan.

For years, I really resented my mum (and dad) for the constant barrage of diet talk and weight-loss interventions. But that changed when I started to learn more about diet culture, and how it's inadvertently passed down from generation to generation. In discovering this, I realised that my parents were just as much of a victim of this as I was, if not more …

DON'T BLAME THE MUMS

My first step towards improving my relationship with my mum was by setting a very simple boundary. At the age of 30, I asked her if she could stop talking to me about whatever new fad diet she was on, as I found it quite triggering. It took a little while for her to get her head around this, but she was really receptive and we got there in the end.

As mentioned briefly a moment ago, I sometimes think my parents' generation were impacted even more severely than my generation by diet culture because, unlike mine, they didn't have the online communities that we now have to lift each other up and call bullshit on toxic messaging.

My mum grew up at a time when waif-like models like Twiggy were on every TV show, in every film and in women's magazine. She was taught by her mum to always be on the hamster wheel of dieting and body hatred, and her mum had been taught the same by hers. The more I thought about this, the more I realised that I never stood a chance of having a positive relationship with my body image from the get-go, because she never did.

About six months after I launched my *Go Love Yourself* body confidence podcast, my mum came over and told me it was really helping her. "It's really changing my life," she said, sat on my sofa with tears in her eyes. "I just always thought I *had* to be on a diet." It was a real breakthrough moment for me.

I now have a lot more empathy and understanding of what she's been through and why she was, and is, the way she is. I think, in turn, that she's learnt a lot about herself and why she feels the way she does, as well as what is and isn't acceptable to say.

If you, like me, have a complex relationship with your mum (or dad, or any other family member), I would encourage you to initiate a conversation about it. For me, I find empathy a useful tool to help relieve any anger that lingers for past and present comments. Perhaps it can help you too?

Maybe your mum, like mine, was raised thinking that her worth as a person depended on her taking up as little space as possible by weighing less. So having an open dialogue can be really healthy, and it doesn't need to be confrontational. There may be tears, of course, but I would encourage you not to be scared away by this. Instead, be brave and try.

If your mum, or other loved one, is receptive to the discussion that you open up, you might then be able to take the next step by talking through clear boundaries about what you do and don't find it OK to talk about when it comes to your food choices and your body.

RAISING BODY-CONFIDENT KIDS

While I don't have children myself, I'm extremely passionate about making sure the next generation isn't subject to the same mistakes that we were when it comes to body confidence.

Breaking the cycle of diet culture is a process that takes time and effort. It involves unlearning old beliefs and behaviours, and creating new, healthier ones. But, in doing so, we can create a world where body diversity is celebrated, and food is enjoyed without guilt or shame. A world where our worth is not determined by our weight or the size of our bodies.

"We need to teach kids that their bodies are valuable and worthy just the way they are," says Forbes. "We need to show them that they don't need to diet or change their bodies to be happy and healthy."

Let's talk about the importance of body image. Heartbreakingly, studies show that children from as young as three can feel bad about their body. A 2016 survey carried out by the Professional Association for Childcare and Early Years found that 24% of nursery-age children started to have negative feelings about their bodies, like thinking their tummy was too fat or that they had a weird body shape.

We need to be clear about what body image is, and what it isn't. Often, we're told by the industries who profit from us feeling bad about our bodies that if we change the way we look, our body image will improve. But actually, body image is a psychological construct; it's the way we think and feel, which means that it's so much more than just looking in the mirror and liking what you see. As such, people who don't fit into the "ideal beauty" box can still have a strong, positive body image.

When it comes to body image, researchers tend to look at two things – body satisfaction (liking what you see) and body appreciation (where you feel at home in your body and appreciate what it can do). For kids, this can be appreciating how great it feels to run around the park with friends, or how their bodies allow them to live their everyday lives. So boosting such moments of *appreciation* from as early an age as possible is key, so that too much value isn't placed on the way our bodies *look*, which is when things becomes problematic.

"A positive body image can sometimes be seen as a nice-to-have, but it impacts every aspect of a child's mental and physical health," says Forbes. "Poor body image in children can lead to mental health issues and affect academic performance and social interactions. On the other hand, a positive body image promotes numerous health-promoting behaviours, such as a healthy relationship with food, stress management and boundary-setting. It also impacts how kids show up in class, their behaviours, social connections, and how they treat others."

HOW WE DO ENSURE A POSITIVE BODY IMAGE FOR THE FUTURE GENERATIONS?

This is a complex issue, with no one-size-fits-all solution, because everyone is unique. However, there are a few steps we can take to start the process of creating a body-positive environment.

Acknowledge the culture we live in

Firstly, it's essential to recognise the values of the culture we live in, many of which focus on appearance over other traits. As a result of this, we can't totally prevent kids from seeing toxic messaging, because it exists in so many forms. You may have noticed, for example, how in the children's cartoon *Peppa Pig*, Daddy Pig's body is always the punchline of the jokes, or that Disney princesses all tend to have a particular shape. It's from "little" things like this that kids can "learn" from a very young age that fat is "bad" and thin is "good".

Forbes notes: "You can't always protect them [kids] from these things, but you can ... recognise it." As such, she advises us to "Be aware of how diet culture shows up in our day-to-day lives and choose the right language to talk to children about it." She stresses that we can talk to kids from a really young age about what health is, and help them to learn they can engage in health-promoting behaviours without focusing on the objective of changing the shape of their body – "It's about encouraging kids to start asking questions and become critical consumers," she explains.

Watch your own use of language

Even if we *tell* kids that appearance doesn't matter, children will inherently understand the societal value that is often placed on looks. One step we can take to help stop them from falling into the same cycle of potential body shame as us is to avoid perpetuating any negative messages through the words that we ourselves use. We can do this by, for example, moving away from compliments or comments that are in any way based on appearance, whether positive or negative. Forbes suggests that: "Instead, we can focus on character traits or accomplishments."

Another step she suggests we can take is to educate our children about body diversity and the harm caused by body-shaming, talking to them about how every body is unique and deserving of respect. Plus, we can encourage behaviours such as exercise and a healthy relationship with food in a way that is not at all connected to size or appearance – to emphasise that healthy habits are not tied to a specific body type.

What's tricky here is that commenting on people's bodies is so ingrained in our culture. When we see a friend after a long time and we say, with the best of intentions, "You look amazing!", it can unfortunately reinforce the idea that appearance is the most important thing about us – hence the advice to move away from comments like this and towards focusing on *other* positive qualities that make each person unique, whether kindness, humility, humour or whatever else.

When a child is bullied or receives a negative comment about their appearance, it's a natural response to say, "You're not ugly, you're beautiful!" or something similar. However, once again, this can just reinforce the idea that appearance is the most important thing and invalidate the child's feelings. Instead, it would be good to validate their experience of living in a looks-obsessed culture, emphasise that the way we look is not the most important thing and instead focus on being grateful for everything our bodies do for us, such as allowing us to live our lives and do the things we love.

Set a positive example

Children can learn body dissatisfaction from their parents. If you look in the mirror and sigh, or complain about your chunky thighs or stretch marks, your children will hear that and internalise it.

"We need to be the change we want to see in our children." says Forbes. "Role models play an essential role in breaking the cycle of intergenerational diet culture. Parents and grandparents can be powerful influencers in shaping children's beliefs about their bodies and food. This means challenging harmful beliefs and language around food and our bodies, and not commenting negatively on our own appearance."

A 2021 study, published in *Frontiers in Psychology*, found that parents who had more negative attitudes towards their own bodies and who engaged in more dieting behaviours were more likely to have children who reported higher levels of body dissatisfaction and lower levels of self-esteem. Additional studies have shown that children who are more exposed to diet talk are more likely to engage in dieting themselves. A 2015 study in the *International Journal of Eating Disorders* even found that 34% of five-year-old girls were already talking about going on a diet!

So, while I know it's hard, the next time you want to express dissatisfaction with your body or your appearance in general, either stop yourself from doing so or, at the very least, do it out of the earshot of your kid. They'll thank you for it later.

Choose toys wisely

Another thing that affects children's body image is the toys they play with, which have been shown to significantly impact their ideas about identity, the world and their place in it. "Take Action Man and Barbie, for instance, and you'll immediately notice the clear messages about gender roles," says Forbes. "Men are strong and 'heroic', while women are fashion- and beauty-conscious." Barbie and Action Man are perfect examples of this. American toy manufacturer Mattel introduced the iconic Barbie doll in 1959 – a time when women didn't have access to the birth control pill and before they could even have their own credit card.

Barbie's creator, Ruth Handler (who named the doll after her daughter, Barbara), intended for Barbie to be an aspirational toy. She said her whole philosophy of Barbie was that, through the doll, the little girl could be anything she wanted to be. But is that really the case? "Through playing with Barbie dolls, young girls learn that they can aspire to be an astronaut or a doctor, but only if they have white skin, an impossibly tiny waist, long glossy hair, and legs that seem to go on for miles," says Forbes. "The first Black Barbie wasn't introduced until 1980 and even then she had Eurocentric features."

Let's also talk about Barbie's proportions. Her body–fat ratio is so low that many researchers believe she would be unlikely to have periods if she were a real-life human. Furthermore, because of her measurements she'd be entirely incapable of lifting her head and would have to walk on all fours.

One study in 2006 showed that playing with Barbie correlated with girls having lower self-esteem and an increased desire for a thinner body. After Mattel released a curvy Barbie, another study done in 2019 found that girls ages three to ten reported the larger Barbie was the one they wanted to play with the least, showing that the mere presence of diverse body size options isn't really enough to change girls' behaviours or attitudes.

A paper in 2016 reported that playing with Barbie led to an increased internalisation of the thin ideal among girls ages five to eight. The list of studies that show the negative effects linked with Barbie is lengthy and unequivocal. As much as I loved it, the *Barbie* movie that was released in 2023 pretty much brushes this list aside, instead focusing on toxic masculinity and the patriarchy.

If we fast forward to today, we can see that Barbie has undergone a slight makeover. Along with the original thin Barbie, children can now choose between curvy, tall or petite Barbie, and there are also versions of Barbie as a wheelchair user, with alopecia, Down's syndrome and a prosthetic leg. This move towards diversity is a positive step, particularly given that an estimated 100 Barbie dolls are sold every minute. However, in a 2019 study by US researchers that asked a group of 84 girls aged three to ten years old to assign positive or negative traits to the different types of Barbie dolls, the results showed a clear preference for thin bodies among the children. Interestingly, the girls who reported feeling worse about their own bodies showed fewer negative attitudes towards the original (thinner) Barbie. This suggests that the internalised thin ideal runs deep, even at a young age.

So, is it OK for young children to still play with Barbies? "Yes, it's fine for girls and boys to still play with Barbie," says Forbes. "But conversations around the dolls' bodies being unrealistic are critical, as is encouraging kids to play with non-gendered toys."

Encourage a healthy relationship with food
We all know encouraging a healthy relationship with food is crucial for overall wellbeing.

Forbes says the best way to do this is by talking about it in a neutral way in order to make it a "non-issue". Language is powerful, and kids pick up on it quickly. That's why it's crucial we use neutral language and avoid labelling food as "good", "bad" or "sinful". Even the word "treat" isn't great. Food has many benefits beyond just fuelling our bodies, so let's celebrate the cake at a birthday party instead of telling kids it's "bad" or telling them they can only have a tiny bit, because all it does is set them up for an unhealthy relationship with food.

As discussed in Chapter 2, we also need to neutralise the word "fat" and recognise that it's a descriptive, neutral word, not a negative one. If a child uses "fat" as an insult, we can approach the conversation by reminding them that all bodies are good bodies, and that we don't comment on other people's bodies anyway. Fat isn't an inherently bad word, it's just about the context in which it's used.

Another good way to encourage a healthier relationship with food among the next generation is to get kids more involved in growing and preparing food, as well as helping them to recognise when they're hungry or full.

The Satter Division of Responsibility in Feeding (sDOR), an evidence-based approach to feeding kids, developed by family therapist and feeding and eating specialist Ellyn Satter, can be a useful framework for parents to know about when it comes to this. This model recognises that parents are responsible for providing nutritious food options and setting meal and snack times, while children are responsible for how much and whether they eat. By giving children the freedom to choose what and how much they eat, they will learn to regulate their intake based on their hunger and fullness cues. This approach helps children to develop a positive relationship with food and learn to trust their bodies' natural signals.

It's essential to avoid pressurising children to eat more than they want or to "finish their plate". Nagging kids to "eat up" can put pressure on them to eat beyond their hunger and fullness cues, leading to overeating or a lack of trust in their own body's signals. This can also lead to them feeling guilty or ashamed for eating certain foods or not being able to control their intake.

It's also important to remember that all foods can have a place in a diet. This includes sweet treats like chocolate and cake. Restricting children's access to these foods (as many people are tempted to do) can actually make them crave them even more, as, if they feel like they're never allowed to have sweet treats, they may begin to view these foods as "forbidden" and therefore develop an unhealthy relationship with them.

In addition, it's important to remember that children are naturally curious and will want to try all kinds of different foods, including sweet treats. So again, if they're never given the opportunity to try these, they may end up feel like they're missing out and not know how to handle themselves around them when they do eat them. By parents allowing kids to have access to these types of foods, children are more likely to develop a healthy relationship with them, not to binge when they do have access or develop a fear of them. For example, a piece of fruit or a serving of a dessert could be added to a child's plate *alongside* their main meal. This can help children learn to appreciate different tastes and textures and can also help prevent sweets and treats from becoming "special" foods that are only allowed on certain occasions.

WHAT TO DO IF YOU'RE CONCERNED ABOUT YOUR CHILD'S WEIGHT

As a parent, it's natural to want your child to be healthy and happy. But it's important to separate weight from health and also to remember that weight is influenced by many factors. We shouldn't assume that a child in a bigger body has an unhealthy relationship with food or physical activity, just like we shouldn't assume a child in a smaller body is automatically "healthy".

Weighing children and equating a number on the scale with worth or health is not advised as it can really harm self-esteem and even lead to disordered eating. Strategies such as creating food rules or nagging about vegetable consumption can also be counterproductive. Instead, all the research tells us that promoting peace and contentment with your children's bodies can foster healthy behaviours and prevent negative consequences like eating disorders or avoidance of physical activity.

According to writer and campaigner Molly Forbes, the most important thing you can do is to not voice any concerns to your child at all about their appearance. She says, "The best way to raise a body-happy child is for them to feel loved and accepted just as they are. As soon as we start voicing concerns, even if it comes from a place of good intention, it can be hugely detrimental."

Parents often feel a natural instinct to mould their children into being the same as everyone else, but we need to change the culture around this, rather than trying to change our kids' bodies. There are plenty of ways that you can support their health without conflating it with weight.

It's heartbreaking to see children and teens struggling with the effects of weight stigma, so it really is important to address this issue. But, as we know by now, losing weight is not a simple solution to achieving good health, as every body is different and diets do not always work. Instead, improving health outcomes requires us to address not just nutrition but also the mental health, sleep, stress and movement patterns of our kids. Taking a holistic approach is key to promoting the overall wellbeing of children and teenagers, moving beyond the simplistic notion of weight loss as a solution.

ADVOCATING FOR YOUR CHILD

It's essential to advocate for the children in our lives when small talk gets diet-y or people make comments about someone else's weight or appearance. And that can sometimes mean speaking up even if the child isn't yours.

For example, I have lots of nieces and nephews who I'm determined to protect, even if that means taking their parents aside at times, and having a word. I understand that having difficult conversations can be challenging. But they're vital for creating positive change.

Some examples of difficult conversations include:

- Challenging weight stigma from family members at the dinner table
- Being *that* parent or guardian that contacts the school administration if you see a diet ad on the school gates
- Asking your friend not to discuss a celebrity's weight loss or "body transformation" in front of your children

- Refusing to engage in diet talk and/or making an effort to give
  non-appearance-based compliments the next time you catch up
  with friends.

"I'm not suggesting that you need to march around with a megaphone
or start arguments in the school playground," says Forbes. "Nobody likes
being lectured, especially children. Instead, we can appeal to people's
love for our kids and ask them in a direct but compassionate way to be
more careful with their language or topic of conversation.

IT'S NEVER TOO LATE TO START BREAKING THE CYCLE

As you've been reading this chapter, you may have been thinking about
certain choices you've made in the past that you worry may have had
a negative impact on your child or the children in your life. It's OK to
reflect on these decisions and think about ways to improve, but it's also
important to remember we are all products of the culture and society we
grew up in. So please don't be too hard on yourself.

It's only when parents start learning and making changes that it can have
a ripple effect on their kids, and maybe even on their parents too, in
terms of breaking the cycle. It's all about creating a positive and healthy
environment for everyone to thrive in.

Forbes emphasises that it's never too late to start breaking the cycle, and
that every small step counts. She concludes: "With you advocating for
your precious, brilliant, unique child, they have the chance to be truly
body happy. We don't need to ... accept the path we are currently on
towards raising a generation of kids ashamed of their bodies. Change is
possible, and we are part of the solution."

SELF-EMPOWERMENT TASK

Take a little time out for yourself and look back at the letter you wrote to your body at the end of Chapter 1. How does that feel to you now that you've read the rest of the book?

Feel into this question, and then spend a little time writing another letter to your body – this time letting her know just how much your perception of her has changed, how much better you're going to treat her now, and the kind of positive, beautiful relationship that you would like to nurture with her from here on in.

Here's what I wrote to mine, to give you an example.

Dear body,

Thank you for everything you do for me. I'm so sorry about how I've treated you in the past.

I used to see you as something that needed "fixing", something that fell short of the perfect images I saw in magazines and on the TV. And in my pursuit of that, I punished you with some awful fad diets, some extreme workouts and some really cruel thoughts and words. I know now that I was wrong to do this.

I now see how strong you are, and I promise to treat you with respect, kindness and care from here on in.

It's time to break free from the chains of unrealistic expectations, judgements and negativity, and to embrace you for all that you are.

I promise to no longer let other people's unkind judgements hold me back or stop me from doing the things I love. Instead, I promise to nourish you with nutritious foods, move with you in fun ways, say yes to all kinds of exciting experiences, and replace previous hurtful thoughts with words of acceptance, self-compassion and love.

It's time to celebrate the life that we are living together – and enjoy it to the full. So here's to a new chapter. A chapter of self-liberation, self-acceptance, and maybe even self-love …

With love and gratitude,
Laura

Conclusion
What now?

So here we are. You've made it.

You're now armed with loads more knowledge and insight about the forces that might have been making you feel bad about yourself, *and* how to move beyond them.

You can now choose to stop letting the scales determine your value, stop giving money to companies who make money from you not feeling your best, stop obsessing over diet after diet, and start living your life to the full – just as you are – instead.

You now know that your body – with all its wobbles, cellulite, stretch marks, folds, curves, scars and hairy bits – tells a story of a skin well lived in, and that every body is a beautiful body. Perfect in its imperfection.

You know to focus less on what you look like and more on who you are as a person.

You know to speak to yourself – and your body – with more kindness.

And you know that you are worthy of big, amazing, wonderful, extraordinary things.

My hope for you is that, as you've worked through this book, you'll have made some small steps forward, as well as maybe some huge leaps. But please know that it's also normal to experience some setbacks, too.

It's only natural that you might still have bad body-image days, where you think: "Wow, I thought I'd moved beyond that." So please don't beat yourself up, as you're still learning. So am I.

It's hard to undo a lifetime of the harsh and unrealistic beliefs and expectations that Western diet culture has heaped upon us, and it's hard to free yourself from the prison of diet mentality.

But you *can* do it.

Just keep in mind that you are more than your bad days. And you are stronger than you can ever even know.

I believe in you. It's time to start believing in you, too.

Acknowledgements

I've got a whole bunch of amazing people to thank for getting me through this rollercoaster of a book-writing adventure. So here are a few shoutouts:

Mum and dad, I know parts of this book will have been tough to read, but please know how grateful I am for your sacrifices, your guidance and your love. I feel so incredibly lucky to call you my parents and I love you both more than you will ever know. I hope I've made you proud.

Matt, thank you for putting up with my late-night writing and various meltdowns over the past year. I'm so lucky to have you by my side. I might threaten to bury you under the patio on a daily basis, but the truth is I'd be lost without you.

Maria, thank you for being not just an awesome stepmum but a fantastic friend, too. Thank you for teaching me about what's really important, and for all the laughs. I love you.

Beth, my editor extraordinaire. I knew from our first Zoom meet (with you in your bright jumper and the cute bunting behind you) that we'd be friends. How lucky am I to have found someone as passionate about this book as I am.

Louise, my agent, you're the real magic behind the scenes. Your belief in me and this book gave me the boost I needed to make it happen. Thank you.

Lauren, my sounding board, podcast co-host, and all-around cheerleader. Your messages and voicenotes of encouragement have meant the absolute world. Thanks for always being in my corner.

And lastly, to my teachers Miss Hickmock, Miss Dixon, and Mrs Rosenthall – you are the reason I fell in love with storytelling and the arts, and for that I will be forever grateful.

Sources

Andreyeva, T, Puhl, RM & Brownell, KD (2008). Increasing Prevalence of Weight Discrimination. *National Survey of Midlife Development in the United States (MIDUS)*.

Awad, GH et al. (2015). Beauty and Body Image Concerns Among African American College Women. Journal of Black Psychology.

Barnes, RD & Tantleff-Dunn, S (2010). Food for thought: Examining the relationship between food thought suppression and weight-related outcomes. *Eating Behaviours*.

Bell, RA et al. (2005). Portrayals of food practices and exercise behavior in popular American films. Health Communication.

Bennett Shinall, J (2015). Occupational Patterns of Women Categorized as Obese. Vanderbilt University Law School.

Bensley, J et al. (2023). Weight bias among children and parents during very early childhood: A scoping review of the literature. *Appetite*.

Carrard, I et al. (2019). Associations between body dissatisfaction, importance of appearance, and aging anxiety with depression, and appearance-related behaviors in women in mid-life. *Journal of Women & Aging*.

Charlesworth, TES & Banaji, MR (2019). Changing Attitudes About Body Weight: An Analysis of Implicit and Explicit Bias. Harvard University.

Damiano, SR, Paxton, SJ, Wertheim, EH, McLean, SA & Gregg, KJ (2015). Dietary restraint of 5-year-old girls: Associations with internalization of the thin ideal and maternal, media, and peer influences. *International Journal of Eating Disorders*.

Dittmar, H, Halliwell, E & Ive, S (2006). Does Barbie make girls want to be thin? The effect of experimental exposure to images of dolls on the body image of 5- to 8-year-old girls. *Developmental Psychology*.

Dove Self-Esteem Project (2021). Girls' Perceptions of Beauty and Photo Editing.

Dubowitz, H et al. (2008). Identifying children at high risk for a child maltreatment report. *American Journal of Preventive Medicine*.

Durex (2017). Orgasm Disparities Between Genders.

Elinav, E & Segal, E (2015). Personalized Nutrition by Prediction of Glycemic Responses. *Cell*. Weizmann Institute of Science in Israel.

Engeln, R, Shavlik, M & Daly, C (2018). Influence of Fitness Instructors' Comments on Women's Body Satisfaction. *Journal of Clinical Sport Psychology*. Northwestern University.

FairyGodBoss (2017). The Grim Reality of Being a Female Job Seeker. https://d207ibygpg2z1x.cloudfront.net/raw/upload/v1518462741/production/The_Grim_Reality_of_Being_A_Female_Job_Seeker.pdf [accessed 17 August 2023]

Fikkan, JL & Rothblum, ED (2012). Weight bias in employment. *Journal of Vocational Behavior.*

Fildes, A et al. (2015). Lifetime Chances of Reaching a Healthy BMI for Obese Women. *American Journal of Public Health.*

Flegal, KM et al. (2013). Association of all-cause mortality with overweight and obesity using standard body mass index categories: a systematic review and meta-analysis. *Journal of the American Medical Association.*

Flint, B et al. (2016). Obese Individuals' Reduced Likelihood of Employment. *Journal of Applied Psychology.*

Greenberg, BS et al. (2003). Portrayals of Overweight and Obese Individuals on Commercial Television. *Obesity.*

Harriger, JA, Schaefer, LM, Thompson, KJ & Cao, L (2019). You can buy a child a curvy Barbie doll, but you can't make her like it: Young girls' beliefs about Barbie dolls with diverse shapes and sizes. *Body Image.*

Hazzard, VM et al. (2021). Intuitive eating longitudinally predicts better psychological health and lower use of disordered eating behaviors: findings from EAT 2010-2018. *Journal of Nutrition Education and Behavior.*

Hruby, A & Hu FB (2015). The Epidemiology of Obesity: A Big Picture. *International Journal of Epidemiology.*

Judge, TA & Cable, DM (2011). When It Comes to Pay, Do the Thin Win? The Effect of Weight on Pay for Men and Women. *Journal of Applied Psychology.*

Lantz, PM et al. (2005). Stress, life events, and socioeconomic disparities in health: results from the Americans' Changing Lives Study. *Journal of Health and Social Behavior.*

Luppino, FS et al. (2010). Overweight, obesity, and depression: a systematic review and meta-analysis of longitudinal studies. *Obesity.*

Marshall, RD, Latner, JD & Masuda, A (2019). Internalized Weight Bias and Disordered Eating: The Mediating Role of Body Image Avoidance and Drive for Thinness. *International Journal of Eating Disorders.*

McLaren, L & Kuh, D (2008). Body Dissatisfaction in Midlife Women. *Journal of Women & Aging.*

Naumann, E, Biehl, S & Svaldi, J (2019). Eye-tracking study on the effects of happiness and sadness on body dissatisfaction and selective visual attention during mirror exposure in bulimia nervosa. *International Journal of Eating Disorders.*

Oldham-Cooper, RE et al. (2011). Distractions While Eating Increase Amount Consumed. *Journal of Nutrition and Dietetics.*

Petrocchi, N, Ottaviani, C & Couyoumdjian, A (2017). Compassion at the mirror: Exposure to a mirror increases the efficacy of a self-compassion manipulation in enhancing soothing positive affect and heart rate variability. *Journal of Positive Psychology.*

Pop M, Miclea S, Hancu N (2004). The role of thought suppression on eating-related cognitions and eating patterns. *The International Journal of Obesity and Related Metabolic Disorders.*

Professional Association for Childcare and Early Years (PACEY) (2016). Negative Body Image in Nursery-Age Children.

Puhl, RM & Heuer, CA (2010). Obesity Stigma: Important Considerations for Public Health. *American Journal of Public Health.*

Solano-Pinto N et al. (2021). Can Parental Body Dissatisfaction Predict That of Children? A Study on Body Dissatisfaction, Body Mass Index, and Desire to Diet in Children Aged 9-11 and Their Families. *Frontiers in Psychology.*

Striegel-Moore, RH & Franko, DL (2003). Epidemiology of Binge Eating Disorder. *Journal of Eating Disorders.*

Throop, EM et al. (2014). Pass the Popcorn: "Obesogenic" Behaviors and Stigma in Children's Movies. *Obesity.* University of North Carolina.

Tomiyama, AJ et al. (2016). Misclassification of cardiometabolic health when using body mass index categories in NHANES 2005–2012. *International Journal of Obesity.*

Tylka, TL (2006). Development and psychometric evaluation of a measure of intuitive eating. *Journal of Counseling Psychology.*

University of Exeter (2016). Earnings Disparity for Slightly Overweight Women.

Zaccagni, L et al. (2014). Body image and weight perceptions in relation to actual measurements by means of a new index and level of physical activity in Italian university students. *Journal of Translational Medicine.*

Further Reading and Resources

BOOKS

Bacon, Linda, *Health at Every Size: The Surprising Truth About Your Weight* (BenBella Books, 2010)

Elman, Michelle, *The Selfish Romantic* (Welbeck, 2023)

Forbes, Molly, *Body Happy Kids* (Vermillion, 2021)

Gordon, Aubrey, *What We Don't Talk About When We Talk About Fat* (Beacon Press, 2020)

Gordon, Aubrey, *"You Just Need to Lose Weight" and 19 Other Myths About Fat People* (Beacon Press, 2023)

Hagen, Sofie, *Happy Fat* (Fourth Estate, 2019)

Kite, Lindsay and Lexie, *More Than a Body* (Harvest, 2021)

Light, Alex, *You Are Not a Before Picture* (HQ, 2022)

Miller, Kelsey, *Big Girl* (Grand Central Publishing, 2016)

Rye, Tally, Train Happy (Pavilion Books, 2020)

Sole-Smith, Virginia, *Fat Talk* (Ithaka, 2023)

Strings, Sabrina, *Fearing the Black Body* (NYU Press, 2019)

Taylor, Sonya Renee, *The Body Is Not an Apology* (Berrett-Koehler, 2021)

Tribole, Evelyn and Resch, Elyse, *Intuitive Eating: A Revolutionary Anti-Diet Approach* (Essentials, 2020)

Wolf, Naomi, *The Beauty Myth* (Chatto & Windus, 1990)

Wolrich, Joshua, *Food Isn't Medicine* (Vermillion, 2022)

Yeboah, Stephanie, *Fattily Ever After* (Hardie Grant, 2020)

RESOURCES

Below is a selection of general mental health and eating disorder resources. Sadly (and unsurprisingly) there is a distinct lack of support for those that struggle with the issues this book addresses – from breaking free of diet culture and redefining what "health" looks like, to increasing body acceptance, the visibility of body diversity and promoting intuitive movement and eating. I am optimistic that this will change, but for the time being, I hope these resources help.

The Satter Division of Responsibility in Feeding (sDOR) – www.ellynsatterinstitute.org

An evidence-based approach to feeding children developed by family therapist and feeding and eating specialist Ellyn Satter. It can be a useful framework for parents to know about.

UK

Beat – beateatingdisorders.org.uk
Offers information and advice on eating disorders, and runs a supportive online community.

British Association for Behavioural and Cognitive Psychotherapies (BABCP) – babcp.com
Information about cognitive behavioural therapy and related treatments, including details of accredited therapists.

British Association for Counselling and Psychotherapy (BACP) – bacp.co.uk
Professional body for talking therapy and counselling. Provides information and a list of accredited therapists.

Gateway Women – gateway-women.com
A support and advocacy network for childless women.

Hub of Hope – hubofhope.co.uk
UK-wide mental health service database. Lets you search for local, national, peer, community, charity, private and NHS mental health support. You can filter results to find specific kinds of support.

Mind – www.mind.org.uk
0300 123 3393 9am–6pm, Monday–Friday [except bank holidays]
Mental health charity which offers information, advice and local services. Local Minds provide mental health services in communities across England and Wales.

Overeaters Anonymous Great Britain – oagb.org.uk
Local support groups for people with eating issues/disordered eating

Samaritans – samaritans.org

116 123 (freephone)

jo@samaritans.org

Samaritans is a listening service (they don't offer advice) and is open 24/7 for anyone who needs to talk. You can visit some Samaritans branches in person. They also have a Welsh Language Line on 0808 164 0123 (7pm–11pm daily).

Talk ED – talk-ed.org.uk

Advice and support for anyone affected by disordered eating.

Tommy's – tommys.org

Information and support for people affected by stillbirth, miscarriage and premature birth.

USA AND CANADA

Crisis Service Canada – www.ementalhealth.ca

Director of mental health services in Canada

Mental Health America – www.mhanational.org

Mental health information and resources, including local services.

National Eating Disorders Association (NEDA) –

www.nationaleatingdisorders.org

A nonprofit, helping individuals and families. This organization has a crisis text messenger service and helpline.

Project Heal (US, Canada and Australia) – www.theprojectheal.org

Offers support and eating disorder treatment programmes.

AUSTRALIA AND NEW ZEALAND

Beyond Blue – www.beyondblue.org.au
Online mental health support and counselling.

The Butterfly Foundation – butterfly.org.au
Support for eating disorders and body image issues.

Mental Health Foundation of New Zealand – www.mentalhealth.org.nz
Resources, support and education.